RIDING

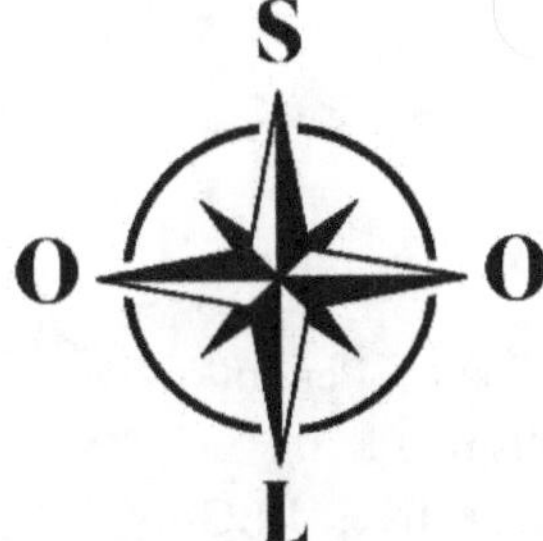

SOLO

A Science-Based Guide to Autonomy, Purpose, and Confidence for Single Women in Midlife

DR. TINA M. PENHOLLOW

ISBN Paperback: 978-1-966018-30-8
ISBN eBook: 978-1-966018-31-5

First edition, 2026

Cover and interior design: Timeless Perspectives Publishing
www.drtinapenhollow.com

Table of Contents

To the Reader:
If you have ever been asked, *"So… are you seeing anyone?"* As if your life were still waiting to begin. Then this book is for you.

.

Introduction

At some point, every woman hears it. Sometimes out loud. Sometimes in silence. A quiet question that lingers longer than it should: "Is this it… or am I still waiting for my real life to begin?"

Your Life is Not a Waiting Room
There is a moment, often quiet and easy to miss, when something shifts. It does not arrive with a dramatic announcement. It does not ask for permission. It appears in ordinary spaces. At the end of a long day. In the stillness of your home. While scrolling through photos of other people's milestones. And it asks a question that feels both unsettling and liberating: *What if this is not a waiting room? What if this is my life?* Not the prelude. Not the rehearsal. Not the space between chapters. This. Right now.

For many women in midlife, this realization changes everything. Because if this is your life, then something is no longer waiting to be completed. It is something already whole. Already unfolding. Already yours.

And yet, despite how full your days may be, there is often an undercurrent, subtle but persistent, suggesting something is missing. Not because it is. But because you were taught to believe it is.

The Story You Were Given

From an early age, most women are handed a script. A quiet but powerful sequence of expectations: Grow up. Fall in love. Build a life with someone. Measure success by partnership. Over time, this script becomes more than a suggestion. It becomes standard. A benchmark. A timeline. A definition of what it means to be "on track." Anything outside of that path is often treated as temporary.

Or worse, incomplete. Single becomes a label. A status. A question waiting to be resolved. "Still single." "You'll find someone." "It will happen when you least expect it." These phrases sound harmless. Even kind. But beneath them lies a powerful assumption: *Your life has not fully arrived yet.* This book challenges that assumption.

A Different Truth

Here is what rarely gets said clearly enough: *Single is not a waiting room.* It is life. A real, valid, meaningful, and often deeply powerful way of living. And increasingly, it is not the exception. It is the reality.

More women than ever are living single in midlife, not as a phase, but as a fully realized way of life. Many discover something unexpected along the way. Not emptiness. Not failure. But clarity. Autonomy. Peace. Strength. A deeper alignment between who they are and how they live.

Culture Needs to Catch Up

The dominant narrative still insists that something essential is missing from a woman's life if she is single. It implies that time is slipping away, that independence is only a temporary phase, and that fulfillment remains just out of reach without a partner. This narrative is not only outdated. It is fundamentally inaccurate. More importantly, it is heavy.

It places an invisible burden on women to measure their lives against a standard that no longer reflects reality or the full range of human experience. This book exists to help you release that weight. To question what was handed down. To redefine what it means to live well. And to recognize that a life lived on your own terms is not lacking anything at all.

This is not a book about rejecting love. It is not about independence for its own sake. And it is not about persuading you to remain single. It is about something far more powerful: *Recognizing the strength, agency, and possibility within the life that is already yours.*

What This Book Will Help You Do
- Release inherited expectations about what a "successful" life is supposed to look like
- Strengthen an internal foundation grounded in self-trust and autonomy
- Understand what research reveals about singlehood, health, and well-being
- Reframe time alone as a source of restoration, clarity, and growth
- Expand your definition of love beyond the traditional couple-centered model
- Design a future guided by intention, stability, and personal alignment

This book offers both a shift in perspective and a framework for action. Because awareness, on its own, is not enough. Lasting change occurs when insight is translated into aligned, intentional choices.

The SOLO Method
To bring structure to what may feel scattered or uncertain, this book introduces a guided framework:

The SOLO Method
A model for building a self-authored life in midlife. Life is shaped from within rather than directed by expectation.

- **Sovereign** — Claiming authority over your identity, values, and decisions
- **Ownership** — Taking responsibility for your patterns, choices, and direction
- **Liberated** — Expanding love and connection beyond traditional, couple-centered definitions
- **Outlook** — Designing your future with intention, stability, and clarity

This is not a system to memorize. It is a framework you will begin to recognize. Because at some level, you already understand this truth: *This is your life. And you are allowed to build it in a way that reflects who you are.*

A Final Word Before You Begin
There is nothing wrong with choosing partnership. There is also nothing wrong with choosing yourself. And there is nothing wrong with creating a life where both exist, but on your terms. Because meaning is not found in following someone else's map. It is created in the way you walk your own path.

If a quiet voice within you has ever asked: Is there another way to live this life? *This book is your invitation to explore it.*

Part I: Reclaiming Your Authority

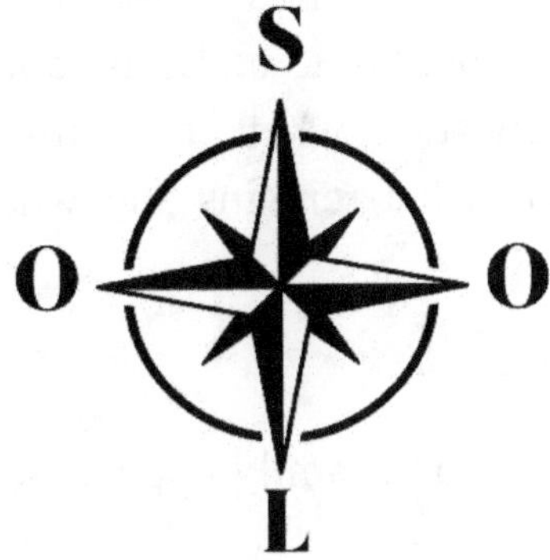

There comes a moment when something no longer fits.

It is not always loud. It does not arrive with a dramatic ending or a clear beginning. It shows up quietly. In a thought that lingers. In a question that refuses to disappear.

Is this really what my life is supposed to look like?

For many women, this moment marks the beginning of something important. Not a breakdown, but recognition. The realization that the life being lived may have been shaped more by expectation than by truth.

Part I is about that recognition. This section introduces the first two elements of the SOLO Method:

- **Sovereign**: reclaiming authority over identity, values, and direction

- **Ownership**: taking responsibility for the beliefs, patterns, and choices shaping your life

Together, these form the foundation of a self-authored life.

In these chapters, the inherited script is examined closely. Not to reject it entirely, but to understand it. To see where it came from. To question whether it still applies. And to consciously decide what remains and what is ready to be released.

You will explore:

- How cultural and family expectations quietly shape decisions

- What science reveals about singlehood and well-being

- Where internal conflict signals misalignment rather than failure

- How to shift from external validation to internal authority

This is not about becoming someone new.

It is about recognizing who has been there all along, beneath the noise.

Because the moment you stop asking, *"What am I supposed to do?"* and begin asking, *"What actually fits me?"*
Something powerful begins.

Chapter 1: The Sovereign Single

Most women are taught, often implicitly, to evaluate their lives through external standards. Family, culture, religion, and media set expectations that quietly position romantic partnership as the central marker of adulthood and success. Over time, these expectations become internalized, shaping decisions long before they are consciously examined. Within the SOLO Method, this chapter establishes the Sovereign dimension, focusing on reclaiming internal authority over identity, values, and life direction.

A single sovereign life begins when these inherited standards are no longer treated as fixed truths, but as one possible narrative among many. The central question shifts: From: *What is expected of me?* To: *What genuinely aligns with the person I am becoming?*

Figure 1 illustrates the SOLO Method: the four interconnected dimensions of a self-directed life. Sovereign establishes internal authority, Ownership reinforces responsibility for choices, Liberated expands definitions of connection and fulfillment, and Outlook provides a forward-focused vision for sustainable well-being.

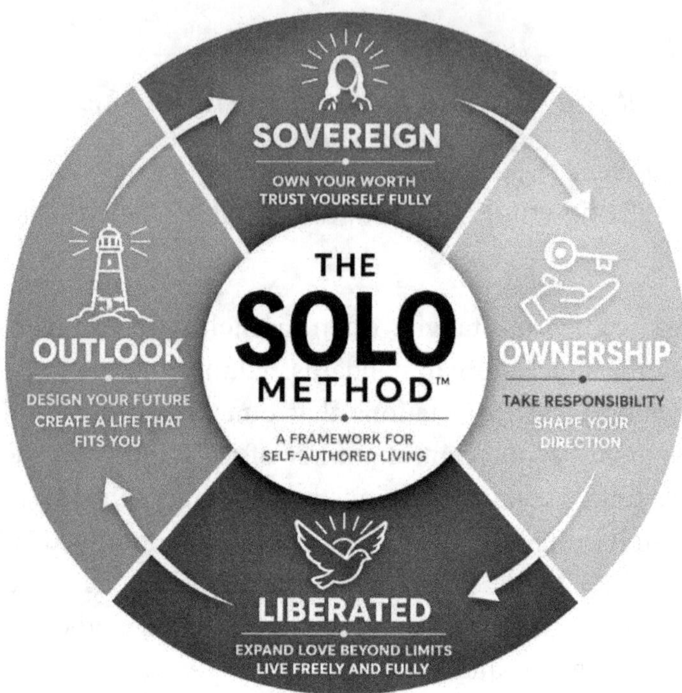

**Figure 1. The SOLO Method:
A Framework for Self-Authored Living**

The Inherited Script

From early childhood, most women are exposed to a culturally reinforced sequence of milestones. Romantic partnership is positioned as the natural and expected destination, with life unfolding along a predictable timeline.

These expectations are rarely presented as optional. Instead, they are embedded in socialization processes across multiple domains: Family narratives and expectations, religious and cultural teachings, media portrayals of relationships, and social reinforcement through peers and institutions.

Over time, repetition transforms these expectations into perceived norms. Behavioral science demonstrates that repeated exposure increases perceived legitimacy, even when the underlying assumption lacks empirical support. This phenomenon, often described as norm internalization, explains why culturally dominant life paths are frequently accepted without critical evaluation.

As a result, deviation from the expected path may feel uncomfortable, not because it is inherently problematic, but because it is less familiar.

The Normalization of Singlehood
Contrary to traditional narratives, long-term singlehood is no longer rare. Demographic data indicate a substantial and growing proportion of women remain unmarried into midlife.

In the United States, approximately one in five women reach age forty without having married, and projections suggest that this proportion will continue to increase (Fry, 2023). These patterns reflect broader social changes, including increased educational attainment, economic independence, and shifting cultural norms.

Importantly, these trends do not indicate relational failure. Instead, they reflect expanded autonomy and the diversification of life pathways (DePaulo, 2017).
Singlehood is not a deviation from adulthood. It is one of several valid expressions of it.

What Sovereignty Means
Sovereignty refers to the capacity for self-governance. In a psychological context, it reflects the ability to regulate behavior, make decisions, and construct a life aligned with personal values rather than external pressure.

For women in midlife, sovereignty represents a critical developmental shift:
- Identity is internally defined
- Decisions are value-driven
- Boundaries are self-determined
- External expectations are evaluated, not obeyed

This is not isolation or disengagement. It is intentional authorship. A sovereign woman may choose to enter a partnership or not. The defining feature is not relationship status, but agency.

Why the Couple-Centered Model Persisted
Historically, romantic partnership functioned as a structural necessity. It provided:
- Economic security
- Social legitimacy
- Division of labor
- Legal and financial protection

For much of history, women's access to resources and autonomy was limited, making partnership essential rather than optional. However, contemporary conditions have shifted significantly. Women now have greater access to:
- Education
- Employment
- Financial independence
- Legal rights

As a result, the function of partnership has changed. It is no longer required for survival or legitimacy. It is one possible component of a meaningful life, rather than its defining feature.

Autonomy and Psychological Well-Being
Self-Determination Theory (SDT) provides a well-established framework for understanding human motivation and well-being. According to SDT, individuals thrive when three core psychological needs are supported:
- **Autonomy**: the ability to make self-directed choices
- **Competence:** experience of effectiveness and growth
- **Relatedness**: meaningful connection with others

These needs can be fulfilled within or outside of romantic partnerships. Research indicates that when individuals experience autonomy, well-being increases regardless of relationship status.

Single women, particularly those who view their status as self-congruent, often report higher self-direction, greater alignment between values and behavior, stronger emotional independence, and higher levels of personal mastery (DePaulo, 2023; Girme et al., 2023).

The Hidden Influence of Social Language
Cultural expectations are often reinforced through everyday language. Phrases such as: "Still single," "You'll find someone," or "When you settle down." Over time, this messaging contributes to a phenomenon known as identity-based pressure, in which individuals feel compelled to align their lives with socially validated roles.

When identity and behavior are misaligned, individuals may experience: Chronic dissatisfaction, low-grade anxiety, and a sense of living inauthentically. These responses are not indicators of personal failure. They signal misalignment between internal values and external expectations.

Reclaiming Authority
Sovereignty begins with recognition. The realization that:
- Not all expectations are personal truths
- Not all cultural norms are evidence-based
- Not all widely accepted paths are universally fulfilling

From this recognition, a shift becomes possible. Instead of adjusting identity to fit the dominant narrative, A sovereign woman adjusts her life to fit her identity. This shift does not require rejecting love, partnership, or connection. It requires removing their status as the sole measure of a meaningful life.

A Different Starting Point
There is no universal path that guarantees fulfillment. There is no single structure that defines success. There is only the question: *What kind of life feels aligned, meaningful, and sustainable for me?* From that question, a different kind of life emerges. One that is not inherited but constructed. Not reactive, but intentional. Not externally validated, but internally grounded.

Integration: Applying the SOLO Method
Use these exercises to begin reclaiming authority over your identity, values, and life direction.

1. Identify the Inherited Script
Write down three beliefs you were taught about what a "successful" life should look like. Next to each belief, ask:
- *Where did this come from?*
- *Do I truly believe this, or have I accepted it without question?*

2. Redefine Your Standard

Complete the following sentence without referencing anyone else's expectations: *A meaningful life, for me, is defined by...* Allow your response to reflect your values, not social norms.

3. Authority Shift Exercise

Notice one recent decision you made. Ask yourself:
- *Was this decision based on expectation or alignment?*
- *What would this decision look like if it were fully self-directed?*

Rewrite the decision from the place of internal authority.

4. Language Awareness Practice

Pay attention to language, both internal and external, over the next few days. Notice phrases such as:
- *"I should..."*
- *"I'm supposed to..."*
- *"At this stage, I need to..."*

For each, pause and ask: *Is this truth, or is this conditioning?*

5. Define Your Sovereign Identity

List 3–5 qualities that define who you are, independent of relationship status, roles, or external validation.

Examples may include:
- Independent thinker
- Creative
- Resilient
- Curious
- Grounded

Then ask: *Am I currently living in alignment with these qualities?*

6. One Aligned Action

Choose one small action this week that reflects your internal authority. This could include setting a boundary. deciding without seeking validation or saying no where you would normally comply. Afterward, reflect: *Did this action feel uncomfortable, or did it feel like clarity?*

Chapter 2: The Weight of Expectation

Expectation is one of the most subtle yet powerful forces shaping your life. It does not arrive as a rule. It rarely announces itself. Instead, it accumulates quietly over time through stories, family conversations, cultural norms, and repeated messages about what a woman's life is "supposed" to look like. Long before these ideas are questioned, they begin to feel natural. Within the SOLO Method, this chapter deepens the Sovereign dimension by examining how external expectations shape identity and influence decision-making.

You may not remember when you first absorbed them, but you are likely to recognize their presence. The assumption that adulthood leads to partnership. The belief that a "complete" life is shared. The quiet pressure that something is missing if it is not.

These messages form what behavioral scientists describe as normative influence, the tendency to align thoughts and behaviors with perceived social expectation. Over time, repetition gives these expectations authority. What is familiar begins to feel true, even when it does not reflect your lived experience.

Within the SOLO Method, recognizing this influence is an act of Sovereign awareness. It is the moment you begin to separate inherited expectations from your own values.

The Script You Were Given
From early childhood, most women are exposed to a culturally reinforced life script. Partnership is positioned not simply as one possibility, but as the central milestone around which everything else is organized. This script is communicated through multiple channels:

- Family narratives and expectations
- Cultural and religious traditions
- Media portrayals of relationships
- Everyday language that frames singlehood as temporary

Individually, these messages may seem insignificant. Collectively, they form a powerful framework that shapes how you evaluate your life. Sociologists refer to this as relationship hegemony, a system in which partnership is treated as the default and preferred state, while other ways of living are viewed as secondary or incomplete (DePaulo, 2017). You may notice how this shows up in subtle ways: "Still single." "You'll find someone." "When you settle down." These phrases are not neutral. They suggest that your life is in transition, even when it is fully formed.

When Expectation and Identity Diverge
When your life aligns with your internal values, there is a sense of coherence. When it does not, something feels off.

Research on identity and motivation consistently shows that well-being is highest when individuals make choices aligned with their core values rather than external pressure (Ryan & Deci, 2020).
When that alignment is missing, the result is often subtle but persistent:

- A low level of restlessness or dissatisfaction

- Irritation in environments where expectations feel strongest
- A sense of performing rather than living
- Resentment toward milestones that never felt personally meaningful

These experiences are not signs that something is wrong with you. They are signals. They indicate that the life being lived may be shaped more by expectation than by intention.

The Changing Reality of Singlehood
Despite persistent cultural narratives, the reality of women's lives has shifted significantly. More women are remaining single into midlife, often by choice or through intentional life design. In the United States, a growing proportion of adults live without a spouse or partner, reflecting broader changes in education, economic independence, and social norms (Fry, 2023).

Importantly, research does not support the assumption that singlehood is inherently associated with poorer well-being. Studies indicate that individuals who experience their single status as self-congruent often report high levels of autonomy, personal growth, and life satisfaction (Girme et al., 2023; DePaulo, 2023). In other words, a meaningful life is not dependent on partnership. It depends on alignment.

Family as the First Influence
For many women, the earliest and most enduring source of expectation is family. Questions that appear harmless can carry weight over time: "Are you seeing anyone?" "You don't want to wait too long." "You deserve someone."

These comments are often rooted in care, not criticism. Yet even well-intentioned messages can reinforce the idea that your life is incomplete without a partner. Because family relationships are emotionally significant, their expectations can feel less like opinions and more like obligations.

Behavioral research shows that the closer the social group, the stronger the influence on decision-making. You may find yourself navigating not only your own desires, but the imagined expectations of the people you care about most.

Reclaiming Your Authority
Sovereignty begins when you pause long enough to ask: *Is this what I truly want, or what I have been taught to want?*

This question is not an act of rebellion. It is an act of clarity. It allows you to: recognize inherited beliefs, evaluate them intentionally, and decide what remains relevant

Reclaiming authority does not require rejecting your family, your culture, or your past. It requires updating the internal framework through which you interpret them. Some expectations may still resonate. Others may no longer fit. Both can be acknowledged without judgment.

From Pressure to Choice
The weight you feel is not failure. It is information. It signals that the story you inherited no longer aligns with the life you are building. As your options expand, so does your definition of a meaningful life. Partnerships are no longer a requirement. It is one choice among many. The question shifts from expectation to alignment. There is often a quiet moment when this becomes clear: *My life already has shape.* It is not waiting to begin. It is already in motion. This is the turning point. The shift from pressure to choice.

Integration: Applying the SOLO Method
Use these exercises to recognize, evaluate, and release expectations that no longer align with your life.

1. Identify External Pressures

Write down three expectations you currently feel about your life. These may relate to:

- Relationships
- Timing ("by now I should…")
- Milestones or roles

Next to each, ask:

- Who does this expectation belong to?
- What happens if I do not meet it?

2. Trace the Origin

Choose one expectation that feels particularly strong. Explore:

- When did I first become aware of this belief?
- Was it explicitly stated or subtly reinforced?
- Does it reflect my lived experience today?

This exercise separates familiarity from truth.

3. Misalignment Detection

Reflect on a recent situation where you felt:

- Irritated
- Pressured
- Slightly "off"

Write:

- What was expected of you
- What you actually wanted

Then ask: *Was the discomfort coming from the situation, or the expectation attached to it?*

4. Language Reframe

Notice how expectation appears in everyday language.

Write down three phrases you've heard or said:

- "You'll find someone."
- "You don't want to wait too long."

- "When you settle down."

Now rewrite each in neutral or self-directed language.
Example: Instead of → "I should be in a relationship by now." Rewrite → "I am choosing the relationships that align with my life."

5. Separate Expectation from Identity
Create two columns:
Column 1: What Is Expected of Me
Column 2: What Actually Fits Me
List freely. Then review:
- Where are they aligned?
- Where are they clearly different?

This is where clarity begins.

6. Redefine Choice
Complete the sentence: *If expectation were removed, I would choose…*
Do not filter for practicality or approval. Focus only on alignment.

7. One Release Action
Choose one expectation you are ready to loosen this week. This does not require a dramatic change. It may be:
- Not explaining your choices
- Not correcting someone's assumption
- Choosing differently in a small moment

Afterward, reflect: *Did releasing this create discomfort, or did it create space?*

Chapter 3: What The Science Actually Shows

"Single is how we live our best, most authentic, meaningful, and fulfilling life."
— Bella DePaulo, PhD, Social Psychologist

Reclaiming the Narrative Through Evidence
For decades, cultural narratives about single women have been presented with confidence yet supported by remarkably little evidence. You have likely heard variations of the same assumptions: That single women are lonely. That they are less fulfilled. And that something essential is missing. *Within* the SOLO Method, this chapter strengthens Ownership by grounding your understanding of singlehood in empirical evidence rather than cultural assumptions.

These claims persist not because they are accurate, but because they have been repeated. When you turn to the research, a very different picture emerges. Across psychology, sociology, and public health, evidence consistently shows that single women are not defined by deficit. Instead, many demonstrate high levels of autonomy, emotional resilience, and relational depth. What changes in this chapter is not your life. It is the lens through which you see it.

The Rise of Singlehood: A Structural Shift
You are not an exception. You are part of a broader social transformation.

Across the United States and much of the developed world, the proportion of adults who are unmarried has increased steadily over the past several decades.

Nearly half of U.S. adults are now unmarried, and a significant number live alone or outside of romantic partnerships (Fry, 2023). This shift reflects structural change, not personal failure. Key drivers include:
- Increased educational attainment among women
- Greater financial independence
- Expanded career opportunities
- Longer life expectancy
- Broader cultural acceptance of diverse life paths

As these factors expand, partnership becomes less of a requirement and more of a choice. Sociologists describe this shift as the individualization of adult life, in which women increasingly shape their lives according to personal values rather than inherited roles (DePaulo, 2017).

Well-Being and Psychological Health
One of the most persistent myths you may have internalized is that singlehood leads to loneliness or poor mental health. The data do not support this. Research shows that women who experience their single status as self-congruent often report high levels of (Girme et al., 2023; Park et al., 2022):
- Life satisfaction
- Emotional stability
- Personal growth
- Autonomy

In fact, satisfaction with singlehood often increases after age forty, particularly when your lifestyle aligns with your values rather than external expectations (Park et al., 2022). This distinction matters. It is not relationship status that determines well-being. It is alignment.

Relational Richness: A Different Model of Connection

If you have ever been told that a partner is the primary source of connection, the research suggests a more expansive reality.

Many single women develop what sociologists describe as relational richness (DePaulo, 2017; Girme et al., 2023):

- Broader social networks
- Stronger friendships
- Frequent contact with family and community
- Diverse sources of emotional support
-

Instead of focusing emotional needs on one relationship, you spread them across multiple meaningful connections.

This creates resilience.

It also creates flexibility, allowing relationships to evolve without placing the entire weight of fulfillment on a single person.

The Role of Solitude in Psychological Strength

Another overlooked advantage of singlehood is access to intentional solitude. Research on positive solitude shows that time spent alone, when chosen, supports (Nguyen et al., 2018):

- Emotional regulation
- Cognitive clarity
- Creativity
- Self-reflection
-

For many women, solitude becomes a space for recalibration rather than isolation. It allows you to:

- Think without interruption
- Feel without external influence
- Make decisions that reflect your values

Health and the Reality of Independent Living
The assumption that marriage automatically improves health outcomes is overly simplistic. Research consistently shows that relationship quality, not relationship status, is what matters most (Wright et al., 2023).
- Individuals in high-conflict or unsatisfying relationships experience elevated stress and poorer health outcomes
- Single adults with strong social networks and healthy routines often demonstrate comparable or better well-being
- Independent living is associated with greater behavioral autonomy, including physical activity and self-care

For you, this means: a well-designed independent life can be just as supportive, and sometimes more protective, than remaining in a misaligned partnership.

Aging, Independence, and Longevity
Concerns about "aging alone" are often rooted in outdated assumptions rather than current evidence. Gerontological research shows that many single women (Dixon, 2020):
- Maintain strong social engagement
- Participate in community and volunteer roles
- Continue learning and growing
- Sustain independence in daily living

Longevity is most strongly associated with:
- Meaningful social connection
- Purpose
- Engagement in life

The Myth of Incompleteness
The idea that you are incomplete without a partner is not supported by science. It is a cultural narrative.

Research consistently demonstrates that a meaningful life is shaped by (Ryan & Deci, 2020; DePaulo, 2023):
- Alignment with personal values
- Autonomy in decision-making
- Meaningful relationships (of many forms)
- Purpose and engagement

Completion is not something another person provides. It is something you cultivate.

A New Understanding of Singlehood
When you step back and look at the evidence clearly, a different conclusion emerges: Singlehood is not a deviation from a "correct" path. It is a valid, often highly adaptive way of living. It offers distinct strengths:
- Self-direction
- Emotional resilience
- Relational diversity
- Personal growth
- Freedom to design your life intentionally

This chapter is not an argument that singlehood is superior. It is a correction. A recalibration. A return to what the evidence shows.

Ownership: Integrating the Truth into Your Life
Ownership means more than understanding the data. It means allowing that data to reshape how you see yourself.
It asks you to consider: *What if nothing is missing? What if your life is already structurally sound? What if the only adjustment needed is the story you have been told about it?*

This is where research becomes personal. This is where knowledge becomes freedom.

Integration: Applying the SOLO Method
*Use these exercises to recognize, evaluate, and release
expectations that no longer align with your life.*

1. Rewrite the Narrative
List three beliefs you have held about singlehood.
Next to each, write a research-informed alternative.

2. Map Your Connections
Identify your key relationships across:
- Friendships
- Family
- Community

Choose one small action to strengthen each.

3. Alignment Check
Ask yourself: *Are my current choices guided by expectation
or alignment?*
Identify one adjustment.

4. Practice Intentional Solitude
Schedule time alone for restoration, not distraction.
Reflect on how it affects your clarity and well-being.

5. Define Your Future
Complete this sentence: *A successful life, for me, looks
like…*
Return to it when external expectations begin to shape your
thinking.

Chapter 4: Questioning the Script

When You Begin to Question What You Were Taught
At some point, you may notice that the life you were taught to want does not fully match the life that feels right to you. This realization rarely arrives dramatically.
It appears quietly:
- In a moment of hesitation
- In a sense of emotional disconnection
- In a question that lingers longer than expected

Is this what I want? For many women, this question marks a turning point. Not a rejection of everything you have been taught, but a shift toward examining it. Within the SOLO Method, this chapter advances Ownership by identifying misalignment between inherited scripts and internal values.

The Function and Limits of Scripts
Life scripts exist for a reason. They provide structure, predictability, and social validation. They offer a clear sequence of what comes next. But what makes a script efficient also limits it. When a script no longer aligns with your identity, it stops being helpful and begins to feel constrained.

Research in social psychology demonstrates that individuals often rely on descriptive norms, or perceptions of others' behavior, to guide their own behavior (Cialdini & Goldstein, 2004). When most people appear to follow a similar path, that path becomes normalized, even if it is not universally fulfilling. For women, this often takes the form of a relationship-centered script:

- Date
- Commit
- Pick a partner
- Build a life around that partnership

The script is rarely presented as optional. It is presented as expected.

When the Script Stops Fitting
When your internal values diverge from external expectations, you may experience what psychologists refer to as cognitive dissonance. This is the discomfort that arises when your behavior or anticipated choices do not align with your beliefs or identity (Festinger, 1957). For you, this may not feel like a dramatic conflict. It often appears as:

- A sense of relief when plans related to dating fall through
- A quiet resistance to conversations about the "next steps"
- A feeling of performing rather than living
- Unexpected peace in moments of independence

These experiences are not random. They are data. They indicate that the script you have been following may no longer reflect who you are.

Dissonance as Information, Not Failure
Cognitive dissonance is often seen as a problem to be resolved quickly. It can function as a signal for recalibration. When you feel tension between expectation and desire, your mind is identifying a misalignment. Research on identity-based motivation suggests that individuals are more likely to sustain behaviors that feel congruent with their identity and values.

When your actions align with who you are, motivation increases. When they do not, resistance emerges. For you, this means: Discomfort is not a sign you are doing life incorrectly. It is a sign that something requires closer attention.

The Risk of Unquestioned Compliance
Choosing not to question the script can feel safer in the short term. It offers:
- Approval
- Predictability
- Reduced social friction

But over time, unexamined compliance often leads to:
- Diminished sense of agency
- Reduced life satisfaction
- Identity diffusion

Developmental psychologists describe this as living according to externally defined meaning systems, rather than internally constructed ones. In contrast, individuals who transition to self-authorship develop:
- Internal standards for decision-making
- Greater emotional stability
- Stronger alignment between values and behavior

Moving Toward Self-Authorship

Self-authorship represents a shift in how you make decisions. The question changes from: *"What should I want?"* to *"What genuinely aligns with who I am?"* This shift does not occur all at once. It unfolds through small moments of honesty:

- Acknowledging that partnership may not be your primary goal
- Recognizing that independence feels energizing rather than lacking
- Noticing where pressure has been mistaken for desire

Each of these moments strengthens your ability to define your life internally rather than externally.

Rewriting the Narrative

Questioning the script does not require rejecting love, connection, or partnership. It requires removing their status as the default measure of a meaningful life. You are not choosing between:

- Independence or connection
- Autonomy or intimacy

You are choosing how these elements fit into your life. This distinction is critical. It allows you to design a life that includes:

- Meaningful relationships
- Personal autonomy
- Intentional structure

A Moment of Clarity

There is often a quiet moment when this shift becomes clear. Not visible to others. Not necessarily dramatic. Just a steady recognition:

I am allowed to choose differently.
That moment marks the beginning of authorship. It is the point at which your life begins to reflect your values rather than inherited expectations.

Ownership as a Practice
Ownership is not a single decision. It is an ongoing practice. It requires you to:
- Evaluate assumptions
- Notice misalignment
- Adjust over time

This is not always comfortable. It may involve:
- Disappointing others
- Redefining success
- Tolerating uncertainty

Integration: Applying the SOLO Method
Use these exercises to recognize, evaluate, and release expectations that no longer align with your life.

1. Identify Moments of Dissonance
Notice situations that feel slightly off. Write down:
- What happened
- What you felt
- What thought followed

Patterns will begin to emerge.

2. Separate Expectation from Desire
Create two columns: *What I Am Supposed to Want? And What I Actually Want?* Compare them without judgment.

3. Define Your Internal Standard

Ask yourself: *If no one were evaluating my choices, what would I choose?* Write freely for five minutes.

4. Rewrite Your Narrative

Describe a version of your life that reflects your values rather than expectations.
Focus on:
- Daily structure
- Relationships
- Environment
- Priorities

5. Take One Aligned Action

Choose one small behavior that reflects your internal truth.
Afterward, reflect: *Did this bring me closer to myself?*

Part II: Reclaiming Your Life

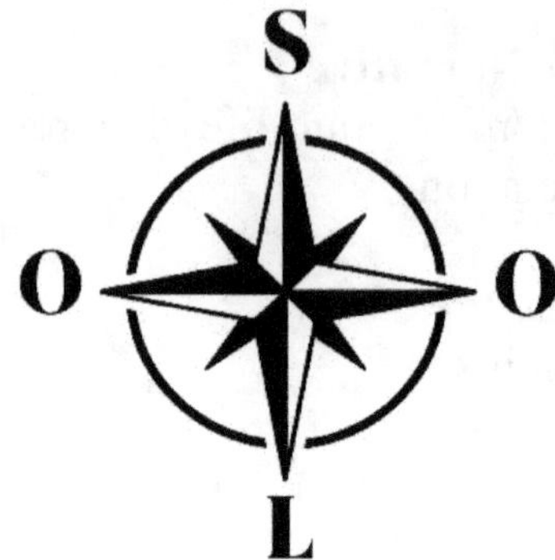

Awareness changes everything. But awareness alone is not enough.

At some point, insight must become action.

Part II marks that shift.

If Part I helped you see the script, Part II asks something deeper:

What does it look like to live differently?

This section moves into the next two elements of the SOLO Method:

- **Liberated** — expanding definitions of love, connection, and fulfillment

- **Outlook** — creating a life that feels stable, intentional, and fully your own

This is where theory becomes lived experience.

Here, singlehood is no longer something to explain. It becomes something to inhabit.

You will explore:

- How autonomy reshapes daily life in quiet but powerful ways

- How solitude transforms from something feared into something restorative

- How relationships can exist outside the traditional couple-centered model

- How purpose, connection, and fulfillment expand beyond expectation

This is not about proving independence. It is about building a life that feels like home. Not someday. Not when something changes. Now.

Because a meaningful life does not begin when someone arrives. It begins the moment you start living it as your own.

Chapter 5: The SOLO Advantage

The Advantage You Were Never Taught to See
Autonomy rarely announces itself in dramatic moments. It reveals itself quietly, in the architecture of everyday life. In how mornings begin. Where energy is invested. Which relationships are nurtured. What is protected, and what is released.

Within the SOLO Method, this chapter reinforces Ownership by examining how autonomy shapes decision-making, behavior, and the structure of daily life. Over time, these small, consistent choices become the foundation of a life that is fully your own.

For many women in midlife, singlehood offers something rarely named with precision: a structural advantage in self-directed living. This advantage is not rooted in the absence of partnership. It is rooted in the presence of authorship. Instead of negotiating identity through constant compromise, life becomes organized around internal alignment. Decisions are not delayed, diluted, or deferred. They are enacted.

Autonomy: A Psychological Necessity, Not a Preference

Autonomy is often misunderstood, particularly for women socialized to prioritize harmony, responsiveness, and relational maintenance. It is frequently mischaracterized as selfishness, rigidity, or emotional distance.

From a scientific perspective, autonomy is none of these. Autonomy refers to the capacity to regulate one's behavior in accordance with internally endorsed values rather than external pressure or expectations (Ryan & Deci, 2020). When autonomy is supported, individuals consistently demonstrate:
- Higher life satisfaction
- Greater psychological well-being
- Improved emotional regulation
- Increased intrinsic motivation
- Enhanced resilience

Internal Locus of Control and the Architecture of Agency
Closely linked to autonomy is the concept of internal locus of control, defined as the belief that life outcomes are shaped primarily by one's own actions rather than external forces. Women with a strong internal locus of control tend to demonstrate:
- Greater adaptive coping
- Lower anxiety and depressive symptoms
- Higher goal attainment
- Increased behavioral consistency

Together, autonomy and internal locus of control create a powerful internal orientation: *I am not waiting for life to happen. I am participating in shaping it.* This orientation is not theoretical. It is behavioral. It is expressed in daily decisions, often without external validation.

Why Singlehood Amplifies Autonomy
Healthy relationships can support autonomy. However, in practice, many women experience subtle erosion of self-direction within couple-centered systems. This erosion rarely occurs through overt control. It occurs through accumulation:
- Coordinated schedules
- Shared priorities
- Emotional negotiation
- Implicit compromise

Over time, individual preferences may become secondary to relational equilibrium. Singlehood disrupts this pattern. It creates a context in which all major life decisions pass through a single internal filter:
- Where to live
- How to structure time
- Which goals to pursue
- How to manage health, finances, and rest
- Who is granted emotional proximity

Research on self-concordant goal pursuit demonstrates that individuals are more likely to sustain behaviors and experience well-being when their actions align with internal values rather than external demands (Sheldon & Elliot, 1999). Singlehood, when lived intentionally, increases the likelihood of that alignment.

Autonomy as a Training Ground for Self-Authorship
Intentional singlehood functions as a developmental environment. It is not merely a lifestyle. It is a context in which self-authorship is practiced repeatedly.

Daily life becomes an ongoing series of decisions that reflect identity rather than expectation:
- Routines align with energy, not obligation
- Work reflects interest, not approval
- Relationships are curated, not inherited
- Rest is protected, not postponed

Research on solitude supports this process. Chosen time alone has been associated with (Nguyen et al., 2018):
- Increased emotional clarity
- Improved decision-making
- Enhanced self-regulation
- Greater cognitive flexibility

The Psychological Cost of Chronic Compromise
Compromise is often framed as a universal virtue. It carries a cumulative cost. Over time, repeated self-adjustment may lead to:
- Identity diffusion
- Reduced intrinsic motivation
- Emotional fatigue
- Subtle resentment

These effects are rarely immediate. They develop gradually through small, repeated concessions. Behavioral research demonstrates that when individuals act in ways misaligned with their values, psychological strain increases (Ryan & Deci, 2020). Autonomy interrupts this pattern. It restores access to internal signals that guide decision-making.

Autonomy and Emotional Health

Autonomy is not only a cognitive construct. It has measurable physiological and psychological effects. When life is guided primarily by external pressure, the body often remains in a low-grade stress response:

- Increased muscle tension
- Disrupted sleep
- Heightened emotional reactivity

As autonomy increases:

- Emotional regulation improves
- Cognitive load decreases
- Stress reactivity diminishes
- Energy becomes available for meaningful pursuits

Research on authentic living indicates that individuals who act in alignment with their core values experience greater well-being and lower psychological distress (Wood et al., 2008). Autonomy is the mechanism through which authenticity becomes behavior.

From Autonomy to Self-Trust

Autonomy establishes structure. Self-trust provides stability within that structure. Self-trust is not confidence in outcomes. It is confidence in one's ability to navigate outcomes. It is the internal recognition:

- I can listen to myself
- I can act on what I hear
- I can respond to what follows

Single living provides repeated opportunities to reinforce this capacity:

- Making independent financial decisions
- Establishing personal boundaries
- Navigating transitions without external direction
- Choosing paths that may not be socially reinforced

Each decision strengthens the feedback loop between autonomy and self-trust. Over time, this loop becomes self-sustaining.

The SOLO Advantage in Relationships
One of the most overlooked outcomes of autonomy is its effect on future relationships. When autonomy is underdeveloped, relationships often become:
- Sources of validation
- Structures of dependency
- Contexts for self-compromise

When autonomy is established, relationships shift fundamentally. They become:
- Voluntary rather than necessary
- Additive rather than foundational
- Aligned rather than compensatory

The internal question changes from: *"Will this relationship complete my life?"* to *"Does this relationship honor the life I have already built?"* This shift is the essence of the SOLO Advantage.

The Presence of Self
Autonomy is not the absence of connection. It is the presence of self. From that position, life becomes:
- Intentional rather than reactive
- Aligned rather than inherited
- Constructed rather than assumed

The SOLO Advantage is not a temporary phase. It is a shift in orientation. A life that is no longer waiting to be validated. A life that is already fully in motion.

Integration: Applying the SOLO Method
Use these exercises to recognize, evaluate, and release expectations that no longer align with your life.

1. Audit Your Daily Structure
Examine how you currently organize your time throughout a typical day. Identify:
  • Where your time feels intentional
  • Where it feels reactive or externally driven
Then ask: *Does my daily structure reflect my priorities, or my obligations?*

2. Autonomy Checkpoint
Reflect on three recent decisions you made. For each, write:
  • What choice did you make
  • What influenced that decision
Then evaluate:
  • Was this decision internally directed or externally shaped?
  • Would I make the same choice again?

3. Identify Energy Alignment
Track your energy over the course of one day. Note:
  • Activities that increase energy
  • Activities that deplete energy
Then ask: *Which parts of my life align with how I function best, and which do not?*

4. Boundary Mapping
List areas where your time, energy, or attention feels overextended. For each, define:
  • What is currently allowed
  • What needs to change
Then complete: *A boundary I need to strengthen is…*

5. Self-Directed Decision Practice

Choose one decision you have been delaying. Without seeking input, complete the following:
- What do I actually want?
- What feels most aligned with my values?

Then act on that decision. Afterward, reflect: *Did acting independently increase clarity or uncertainty?*

6. Strengthen Internal Locus of Control

Write down one area of your life where you feel stuck or uncertain. Then reframe it by identifying:
- What is within your control
- One action you can take immediately

Complete: *A step I can take today is…*

7. One Structural Adjustment

Select one small but meaningful change to your routine this week. Examples may include:
- Adjusting your morning or evening structure
- Protecting uninterrupted time
- Prioritizing a personal goal

After implementing, reflect: *Did this change make my life feel more aligned or more efficient?*

8. Reinforce Self-Trust

At the end of the week, write down three decisions you made independently. For each, note:
- What you chose
- How it felt
- What the outcome was

Then ask: *Am I becoming someone who trusts my own direction?*

Chapter 6: Sacred Solitude

Rewriting What It Means to Be Alone

Time alone is not neutral. It is interpreted. You have likely been taught to see it as an absence. As evidence that something is missing. As a space to fill as quickly as possible. That interpretation is not innate. It is learned. Within the SOLO Method, this chapter reflects Liberated living by redefining solitude as a source of regulation, clarity, and psychological strength.

When solitude is framed as a deficiency, quiet moments feel heavy. When it is understood as intentional space, those same moments become restorative. This chapter asks you to reconsider what you have been taught.

Solitude is not withdrawal from life. It is where your life becomes most visible to you. Within the SOLO Method, this is the essence of Liberated living. You are no longer measuring your life by proximity to others. You are learning to experience it directly.

Solitude and Loneliness: A Critical Distinction

From the outside, solitude and loneliness can look identical. From the inside, they are fundamentally different psychological states.

Loneliness reflects perceived social disconnection. It is associated with increased stress, poorer sleep, inflammation, and reduced well-being (Hawkley & Cacioppo, 2010).

Solitude, when chosen, reflects intentional disengagement for restoration and reflection, a state associated with psychological growth, emotional regulation, and self-reflection (Long & Averill, 2003). It is associated with emotional regulation, cognitive clarity, creativity, and self-awareness (Nguyen et al., 2018).

The difference is not the presence or absence of people. It is whether your time alone is imposed or chosen. When solitude is chosen, it becomes regulation rather than deprivation.

Why Solitude Feels Uncomfortable at First
If quiet feels unfamiliar, that response is not a flaw. It is conditioning. You have likely been immersed in environments where:
- Noise is constant
- Attention is fragmented
- Validation is external
- Distraction is immediate

When those inputs are removed, your internal world becomes more audible. At first, this may feel uncomfortable. Thoughts surface. Emotions intensify. Old narratives replay. This is not a sign that solitude is harmful. It is a sign that you are finally hearing what has been competing for attention. Over time, the experience shifts. What initially feels like exposure becomes clarity.

Solitude as a Regulatory System
Solitude is not simply psychological. It is physiological. When you move away from constant stimulation, the nervous system begins to recalibrate. Heart rate slows. Cortisol levels decrease. Cognitive load reduces.
Research in affective science demonstrates that chosen solitude supports self-regulation, allowing individuals to process emotional experiences more effectively (Nguyen et al., 2018). You begin to notice:
- Your thoughts are less reactive
- Your emotional responses are more proportional
- Your decisions feel less urgent and more deliberate

Solitude becomes a regulatory environment. It is where your system resets.

The Cognitive Function of Solitude
Beyond regulation, solitude enhances cognitive processing. Without continuous external input, the brain engages in what is often referred to as default mode activity, associated with:
- Self-reflection
- Meaning making
- Future planning
- Identity integration

In practical terms, this means:
- Patterns become visible
- Decisions become clearer
- Priorities reorganize

You begin to distinguish between:
- What you were taught to want
- What you want

Solitude as a Site of Identity Formation
Identity is not formed in constant interaction. It is clarified in stillness. When your environment is quiet, you stop responding. You are observing. You notice:
- What energizes you
- What drains you
- What feels aligned

Research on identity-based motivation suggests that behavior becomes more sustainable when it reflects internal identity rather than external expectation. Solitude provides the conditions for that alignment to emerge.

Resilience Is Built in Quiet Moments
Resilience is often misunderstood as endurance. It is more accurately described as adaptive regulation under stress. Solitude supports this process. When you spend intentional time alone, you develop:
- Emotional regulation
- Cognitive flexibility
- Meaning-making capacity

These three components are consistently associated with resilience. In solitude, you are able to:
- Process emotional experiences without interruption
- Reframe situations with greater clarity
- Integrate experiences into a coherent narrative

From Reactivity to Observation
One of the most significant shifts that occurs in solitude is the transition from reactivity to observation. Instead of being immersed in your thoughts, you begin to notice them. Instead of: *"I am overwhelmed."* The shift becomes: *"I am noticing thoughts of overwhelm."*

This distinction, central to mindfulness-based approaches, reduces emotional reactivity and increases behavioral flexibility. You are no longer inside the storm. You are observing it. That shift creates choice.

Solitude and Self-Trust
Solitude regulates and clarifies. It strengthens self-trust. You begin to internalize a critical message: *I can rely on myself.*
Self-trust develops through repeated evidence. Each time you remain present in your own experience without escaping it, that evidence accumulates. Over time, your internal voice becomes clearer, more stable, and more authoritative. This is not confidence based on outcomes. It is confidence based on self-reliance.

Creating an Internal Home
There is a difference between having a place to live and having a place within yourself that feels stable. Solitude allows you to build that internal structure. An internal home is characterized by emotional safety, psychological stability, self-compassion, and consistent self-attunement.

Research on self-compassion shows that individuals who respond to themselves with understanding rather than self-criticism tend to experience lower anxiety, greater psychological resilience, and more effective emotional regulation (Neff, 2011). This kind of internal environment does not arise by chance; it is intentionally cultivated through consistent, mindful attention to one's thoughts, emotions, and needs. Over time, this practice reshapes the way challenges are interpreted and managed, creating a more stable and supportive psychological foundation.

In this process, individuals begin to engage in a more reflective internal dialogue, asking themselves questions such as what is needed in the present moment, what actions or conditions genuinely support well-being, and what choices feel most aligned with their values and sense of self.

Sacred solitude exerts a powerful influence on how relationships are perceived and experienced. When emotional clarity, internal stability, and a self-directed sense of calm become familiar states, a new internal reference point emerges. There is a clear understanding of what it feels like to be regulated, respected, and at ease. This awareness naturally recalibrates relational standards. Tolerance for chronic chaos, emotional volatility, or disregard for time and boundaries begins to diminish, not as a defensive reaction, but because of heightened clarity and self-alignment. Solitude, in this context, does not function as isolation; it serves as calibration, refining expectations and reinforcing what is acceptable and sustainable in interpersonal dynamics.

At the same time, this perspective challenges long-held cultural assumptions about being alone. Many have been conditioned to believe that solitude signals absence, that silence should be avoided, or that personal value is reflected in the constant presence of others. A more accurate and empowering framework recognizes solitude as a regulatory space where the nervous system stabilizes, a cognitive environment that supports deeper processing, and a critical setting for identity clarification. It becomes a foundation for resilience and a direct pathway to strengthening self-trust, allowing individuals to engage with others from a position of clarity rather than dependency.

Integration: Applying the SOLO Method
Use these exercises to recognize, evaluate, and release expectations that no longer align with your life.

1. Redefine Your Experience of Solitude
Write down your immediate associations with being alone.
Then ask: *Do I interpret solitude as absence or as space? Where did this interpretation originate?* Rewrite your definition: *Solitude, for me, is…*

2. Distinguish Solitude from Loneliness
Reflect on a recent moment when you were alone.
Identify: What you felt and what you thought about that feeling. Then ask: *Was this loneliness (disconnection) or solitude (chosen space)?* This distinction builds psychological clarity.

3. Schedule Intentional Solitude
Set aside a specific block of uninterrupted time this week.
During this time: No phone, no media, and no external input
Simply observe: Thoughts, emotions, and your physical state
Afterward, reflect: *What became clearer when the distraction was removed?*

4. Internal Awareness Practice
During a quiet moment, ask yourself:
- *What am I feeling right now?*
- *What do I need in this moment?*
- *What is asking for attention?*

Write your responses without filtering. This builds self-attunement, a core component of Liberated living.

5. Cognitive Clarity Exercise
Use solitude to think through one decision or situation.
Instead of reacting, write: *What are the facts? What assumptions am I making? What matters here?*
Then ask: *What calm, aligned version of me would choose?*

6. Emotional Regulation Check
Notice your emotional state before and after time alone.
Track: stress level, mental clarity, and emotional intensity
Then evaluate: *Does intentional solitude regulate or destabilize my internal state?*

7. Build an Internal Home
List what makes you feel: Safe, grounded, and mentally clear. Then identify: *How can I create these conditions for myself, independently?* Complete: *I create stability in my life by...*

8. One Solitude Ritual
Design a repeatable practice that anchors your time alone.
Examples:
- Morning reflection
- Evening decompression
- Quiet walk without stimulation

Commit to practicing it consistently this week. Afterward, reflect: *Did this make solitude feel more structured and supportive?*

Chapter 7: Love Beyond the Couple

"Women are becoming the men we wanted to marry."
— Gloria Steinem, Writer and Activist

Expanding the Definition of Love

Most relationship models you have been exposed to follow a predictable structure. A romantic partnership sits at the center, and every other connection is organized around it. This model is not neutral. It is cultural. It teaches you to prioritize one form of love while minimizing others.

It suggests that fulfillment is concentrated in a single relationship rather than distributed across many. Within the SOLO Method, this chapter expands the Liberated dimension by redefining love as a distributed system rather than a single relational structure.

This framework is incomplete. Love has never been confined to one relationship. It exists across multiple domains of your life: friendship, community, mentorship, family, purpose, and the relationship you maintain with yourself. When you release the assumption that one person must serve as your emotional center, something shifts. Love expands. You are no longer organizing your life around a single relational axis. You are expanding your capacity to give, receive, and recognize connection in multiple forms.

The Cultural Narrowing of Love

Modern Western culture has elevated romantic partnership to a dominant position. This framework, often reinforced through media, social norms, and institutional structures, suggests that romantic love is primary and that other relationships are secondary. This assumption reflects what scholars describe as *amatonormativity*, the belief that a central romantic relationship is necessary for a complete life (Brake, 2012). You have likely encountered this model repeatedly. It appears in:
- Media narratives
- Social expectations
- Institutional policies
- Everyday language

The underlying message is consistent: a meaningful life is built around a romantic pair. Yet empirical evidence does not support this hierarchy. Human well-being is not dependent on one relationship. It is supported by relational diversity.

The Science of Relational Diversity
You are not designed to rely on one person to meet every emotional, intellectual, and social need. Humans function best within multi-layered relational systems.

Research across psychology, sociology, and public health consistently demonstrates that individuals embedded in diverse social networks experience (Holt-Lunstad et al., 2010; Umberson & Karas Montez, 2010):
- Lower mortality risk
- Reduced chronic stress
- Improved immune functioning

This is not about having more relationships. It is about having varied relationships. Each connection serves a distinct function. One person offers emotional depth.

Another provides intellectual stimulation. Another brings humor. Another offers stability or perspective. Together, these relationships form a distributed support system. This system is often more resilient than a single relational anchor. Connection is not strengthened by concentration. It is strengthened by distribution.

Flattening the Hierarchy of Love
Culturally, relationships are often organized hierarchically. Romantic partners are placed at the top, followed by children, family, and then friends or community. This hierarchy is not evidence-based. It is socially constructed. When you accept this structure, you may unconsciously devalue:
- Deep friendships
- Long-term community ties
- Mentorship relationships
- Chosen family

Reframing begins by flattening this hierarchy. Love is not ranked. It is expressed. A life rich in connection may include:
- Friends who function as family
- Communities that provide belonging
- Mentoring relationships that span generations
- Shared purpose through work, service, or creativity

Research on social integration consistently shows that perceived relational quality, not relationship type, is the strongest predictor of well-being (Umberson & Karas Montez, 2010). The question is no longer: *Do you have a partner?* The question becomes: *Are your relationships meaningful, reciprocal, and aligned?*

Reimagining Family
Family is often treated as fixed. In reality, it is both inherited and constructed. For women in midlife, this distinction becomes increasingly important.

A biological family may provide support, history, and connection. It may also include misalignment, conflict, or emotional strain. Research on adult development shows that individuals actively construct relational ecosystems that support their well-being over time (Antonucci et al., 2014). This includes what is often referred to as chosen family. These relationships are defined not by obligation, but by:
- Mutual care
- Consistent presence
- Emotional investment
- Shared responsibility

These relationships are not secondary. They are adaptive. They reflect intentional connection rather than inherited structure.

The Many Forms of Love in Your Life
When you begin to look more closely, you may already see that your life contains multiple expressions of love. Friendship provides depth, continuity, and emotional safety. Longitudinal research shows that high-quality friendships are strongly associated with well-being across adulthood (Demir et al., 2012).

Community offers shared meaning and belonging. Environments where you feel seen and valued reinforce psychological stability and connection.
Mentorship and intergenerational relationships provide both direction and continuity. These connections strengthen

identity and support long-term development (Feeney & Collins, 2015).

Self-love functions as the structural foundation. It is not indulgence. It is the consistent practice of respecting your limits, honoring your needs, and maintaining boundaries. Research on self-compassion demonstrates that individuals who treat themselves with understanding experience greater resilience and emotional regulation (Neff, 2011). Each form of love serves a distinct function. Together, they create a system.

The Risk of Centralizing Love

When love is concentrated in a single relationship, expectations increase. One person is expected to provide emotional support, validation, companionship, and identity reinforcement. No single relationship can meet all emotional needs. When this expectation is placed on one person, it often leads to:

- Relational strain
- Emotional dependency
- Reduced resilience

Relationship science consistently demonstrates that diversification is adaptive (Feeney & Collins, 2015).

When love is distributed, pressure decreases. Each relationship becomes more authentic. Emotional needs are met across multiple channels. Your sense of belonging becomes more stable. You are no longer asking, "Who will meet all my needs?" You begin by asking: *How is love already present in my life?*

Relational Agency

Expanding your relational world requires agency. You are no longer waiting for connection to happen. You are designing it. Relational agency involves initiating contact, maintaining meaningful ties, creating recurring structures for connection, and setting boundaries that protect emotional capacity.

Individuals who actively maintain relationships report higher levels of satisfaction and connection (Feeney & Collins, 2015). Connection is not passive. It is constructed.

Relational Standards in a Self-Authored Life

As your relational framework expands, your standards shift. This shift does not emerge from rigidity. It emerges from clarity. You become less willing to tolerate one-sided relationships, emotional inconsistency, or lack of reciprocity. Not from defensiveness, but from recognition. You understand what connection feels like when it is mutual, stable, and aligned.

Research consistently shows that perceived equity, responsiveness, and emotional reliability are central predictors of relationship satisfaction and psychological health (Reis et al., 2004; Feeney & Collins, 2015).

When these elements are absent, strain accumulates. When they are present, the connection stabilizes.

You Are Not Lacking Love

One of the most persistent cultural myths is that without a romantic partner, you are less loved. This is not supported by evidence. It is a narrative.

If you look closely, you may already see:

- People who show up consistently
- Relationships that provide support
- Moments of care woven into your daily life

These are not minor interactions. They are expressions of love. The shift is not in acquiring more love. It is in recognizing the love that already exists.

Love as a Distributed System
Love is not a destination. It is a system. When you expand your definition of love:
- Your relationships deepen
- Your sense of belonging increases
- Your life becomes more emotionally stable

A romantic partnership becomes one form of connection among many. Not the measure of your worth. Love is multi-dimensional, system-based, and behaviorally expressed through consistency, attention, care, and reciprocity.

Love Is Already Here
You are not waiting for love to arrive. You are already living within it. When you let go of the idea that love must be centralized, something expands. Your life becomes more connected, not less. More stable, not less. More aligned, not less. This is not a rejection of partnership. It is a reorganization of meaning. Love is no longer something you wait to receive. It is something you recognize, cultivate, and experience across your life.

Love is not a destination. It is a system. When the definition of love expands, relationships deepen, the sense of belonging increases, and life becomes more emotionally stable. A romantic partnership becomes one form of connection among many, not the measure of worth. Love is multi-dimensional, system-based, and expressed through consistency, attention, care, and reciprocity.

You are not waiting for love to arrive. You are already living within it. When the expectation that love must be centralized begins to dissolve, something expands. Life becomes more connected, more stable, and more aligned.

This is not a rejection of partnership. It is a reorganization of meaning. Love is no longer something to wait for; it becomes something to recognize, cultivate, and experience across the full architecture of daily life. What becomes clear is this: the quality of life is not determined by the presence of a single relationship, but by the strength and diversity of a relational ecosystem. When love is distributed, it becomes more resilient, more accessible, and more sustainable over time, no longer fragile or conditional but reinforced across multiple points of connection. This shift returns you to the center of your own life, not as someone waiting to be chosen, but as someone actively creating, maintaining, and recognizing meaningful connection. You are not outside of love. You are operating within it, shaping it, and expanding it through the way you live, relate, and show up each day.

Integration: Applying the SOLO Method
Use these exercises to recognize, evaluate, and release expectations that no longer align with your life.

1. Map Your Relational Ecosystem
List the key relationships currently in your life across: Friendship, family, community, and mentorship. Ask: *Where is the connection present that I may have been overlooking?*

2. Redefine Love
Complete the sentence: *Love in my life is expressed through...* Focus on actions, consistency, and presence rather than roles or labels.

3. One Intentional Connection
Choose one relationship to strengthen this week. Take one small action: Reach out, schedule time, and express

appreciation. Afterward, reflect: *Did this deepen my sense of connection without relying on one central relationship?*

Chapter 8: Purpose Without Permission

"The most courageous act is still to think for yourself. Aloud."
— Coco Chanel, Designer and Entrepreneur

Reclaiming Purpose on Your Terms
You were likely taught that purpose follows a script. Education. Career. Partnership. Children. Stability. Within that sequence, purpose is often implied rather than explored. It is assumed to emerge through socially recognized, externally validated roles.

When your life does not follow that sequence, or no longer feels aligned with it, your sense of purpose can feel uncertain. You may wonder:
- *Am I behind?*
- *Did I miss something?*
- *Does purpose require a specific role?*

These questions are not personal failures. They are the result of a narrow cultural model. Purpose is not assigned. It is constructed through alignment.

Within the SOLO Method, this chapter introduces Outlook by guiding the development of purpose as a self-directed and evolving structure. You are no longer waiting for your life to be validated. You are actively shaping it based on what matters to you.

The Myth of Permission

Many women are conditioned to seek approval before fully engaging with their own lives. Permission may take subtle forms:

- Waiting for the "right time"
- Seeking validation from others
- Aligning decisions with expected roles
- Deferring goals until circumstances feel ideal

This pattern delays action. Research in self-determination theory demonstrates that behavior aligned with internal values, rather than external approval, is associated with higher well-being, persistence, and life satisfaction (Ryan & Deci, 2020). Purpose does not require consensus. It requires clarity.

How Independence Clarifies Direction

When your life is not organized around another person's trajectory, something becomes available. Space. In that space, different questions begin to surface:

- *How do you want to spend your time?*
- *What feels meaningful, even without recognition?*
- *Where does your attention naturally return?*

These questions are not abstract. They are diagnostic. Research on identity-based motivation suggests that behavior becomes more consistent when it reflects internal identity rather than external expectation (Oyserman, 2009). Without constant negotiation, you are able to observe:

- What energizes you
- What depletes you
- What sustains your attention over time

Purpose Is Not a Job Title

One of the most limiting beliefs about purpose is that it must be singular and career-based. This belief is incomplete.

Purpose is better understood as direction, not position. It is expressed through patterns: what you return to, what you invest in, and what you consistently care about. These patterns may appear across multiple domains:
- Work
- Creative expression
- Relationships
- Community involvement
- Personal practices

Research in positive psychology indicates that individuals with a strong sense of purpose demonstrate higher life satisfaction and greater resilience, regardless of occupational status (Hill et al., 2016). Your purpose is not confined to one role. It is reflected in how you live.

The Health Impact of Purpose
Purpose is not only psychological. It is physiological. Longitudinal studies show that individuals with a clear sense of purpose experience (Hill & Turiano, 2014; Kim et al., 2019):
- Lower risk of mortality
- Reduced cognitive decline
- Better cardiovascular health
- Improved emotional well-being

Purpose functions as a regulatory anchor. When circumstances shift, purpose provides continuity. For you, this means: Even when your life does not match expected milestones, it can remain deeply meaningful.

Purpose as Iteration, Not Discovery
Purpose is often framed as something you find once. This framing is inaccurate. Purpose is iterative. It develops through exploration, experimentation, feedback, and adjustment.

Behavioral research shows that individuals who engage in goal exploration are more likely to develop sustained motivation and clarity over time (Sheldon & Elliot, 1999). You do not need a complete plan. You need a starting point.

Letting Go of External Metrics
Cultural definitions of success often rely on visible markers:
- Relationship status
- Income
- Titles
- Social approval

Research on well-being consistently shows that subjective meaning, rather than external achievement, is the strongest predictor of life satisfaction (Steger, 2012). You are not required to meet external benchmarks to live a meaningful life.

You Are Allowed to Begin Now
Purpose is often delayed by the belief that conditions must be optimal. They do not. You do not need more time, more certainty, or more approval. You need movement. Even small actions provide information of what you want.

From Permission to Ownership
The shift from permission to ownership is fundamental. Instead of asking: *"Is this allowed?"* You begin asking: *"Is this aligned?"* This shift changes decision-making. You are no longer organizing your life around expectations. You are organizing it around values. This is the transition from external validation to internal authority.

Integration: Applying the SOLO Method
Use these exercises to recognize, evaluate, and release expectations that no longer align with your life.

1. Redefine Purpose on Your Terms
Write down your current definition of purpose. Then ask: *Is this definition based on roles, achievements, or alignment? Does it reflect what matters to me, or what is expected of me? Purpose, for me, is…*

2. Identify Patterns of Meaning
Reflect on your recent experiences. Identify:
* What consistently holds your attention
* What feels meaningful, even without recognition
* What you return to naturally

Then ask: *What do these patterns suggest about what matters to me?*

3. Remove the Need for Permission
Think of one goal, idea, or direction you have delayed. Ask:
* What am I waiting for?
* Whose approval feels necessary?

Then reframe: *If permission were not required, I would begin by…*

4. Clarify Direction, Not Destination
Write down one area of your life where you want greater purpose. Instead of defining a final outcome, identify: The direction you want to move toward and the type of experience you want to create. Then ask: *What is one step that moves me in that direction?*

5. Align Action with Values
List your top 3 values. For each, write: One behavior that reflects this value in daily life. Then evaluate: *Is my current life structured around what I say matters most?*

6. Release External Metrics
Write down one standard of success you have been measuring yourself against. Then ask:
- Does this standard reflect my values or social expectations?
- What would success look like if it were internally defined?

Rewrite: *Success, for me, now looks like…*

7. One Purpose-Driven Action
Choose one small action aligned with what feels meaningful to you. This could include: Starting something you have postponed, re-engaging with an interest, and taking a step without certainty. Afterward, reflect: *Did acting create clarity or reduce it?*

8. Build Momentum Through Iteration
At the end of the week, write: One action you took, what you learned from it, and what you want to adjust next. Then ask: *Am I waiting to feel ready, or am I becoming ready through action?*

Part III: Designing a Powerful Future

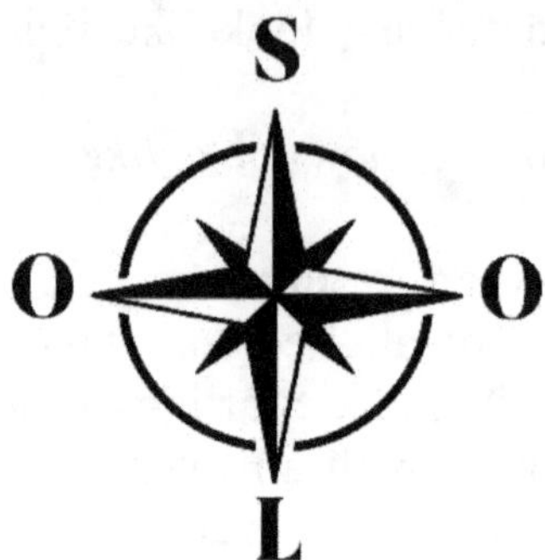

Once a life is reclaimed, a new question naturally emerges: *What do I want to build from here?*

Part III looks forward. This section brings together everything you have explored and turns it toward the future. Not as something uncertain or dependent on circumstance, but as something you are actively shaping.

Here, the SOLO Method becomes fully integrated.
- Sovereign becomes identity
- Ownership becomes responsibility
- Liberated becomes freedom
- Outlook becomes direction

Together, they form a life that is not reactive but designed. You will explore:
- How singlehood influences long-term health, aging, and well-being
- How to navigate moments of doubt without abandoning self-trust

- How to strengthen identity in a culture that still questions it
- How to create a future defined by intention, not expectation

This is where independence becomes power. Not loud. Not performative. Steady. The goal is to build a life so aligned, so grounded, and so fully your own that relationship status becomes secondary to something far more important: the quality of the life you are living.

Chapter 9: Health Benefits of Solo Living

Health Is Not Determined by Relationship Status
For decades, a single idea has shaped how women evaluate their health: that marriage is inherently protective. This belief has been repeated so often that it has come to feel like evidence. Yet contemporary research presents a far more precise conclusion. Health is not determined by marital status. It is determined by alignment. Alignment between your behaviors and your needs. Between your environment and your nervous system. Between your values and how you live each day.

Within the SOLO Method, this chapter applies Outlook as a framework for aligning daily life with long-term physical and psychological health. It shifts the question from *"Am I doing life correctly?"* to *"Is the way I am living supporting my body, mind, and long-term well-being?"* Increasingly, the evidence shows that many women living independently are not merely maintaining health. They are optimizing it.

Autonomy as a Health Mechanism
Autonomy is not only a psychological construct. It is a physiological advantage. Autonomy reduces chronic stress activation, improves emotional regulation, and increases adherence to health-promoting behaviors.
In practical terms, when your life is self-directed:

- Daily routines reflect your biological rhythms
- Health decisions are proactive rather than reactive
- Energy is allocated intentionally rather than negotiated

Physical Health: Living in Synchrony with Your Body
Independent living allows health behaviors to align more closely with physiological needs rather than shared compromise. Research indicates that single adults often demonstrate:
- Higher levels of daily physical activity
- More consistent routines
- Greater engagement in preventive care
- Increased behavioral autonomy in nutrition and sleep

When controlling for socioeconomic status and baseline health, many previously reported "marriage advantages" diminish substantially (Musick & Bumpass, 2012; Wright et al., 2023). In some populations, single women report:
- Lower body mass index
- Greater mobility and daily movement
- More frequent use of preventive healthcare services

The mechanism is straightforward. When decisions are not filtered through another person's schedule or preferences, adherence improves. The body is no longer negotiated with. It is listened to.

Stress, Emotional Load, and Psychological Stability
One of the most persistent misconceptions is that partnership reduces stress. The evidence does not support this as a universal truth. Relationship quality, not relationship status, is the primary determinant of emotional health (Kiecolt-Glaser & Newton, 2001).
High-conflict or misaligned relationships are associated with:

- Elevated cortisol levels
- Increased inflammation
- Greater depressive symptoms
- Reduced immune functioning

In contrast, single adults with strong social networks often report:
- Lower chronic stress
- Greater emotional stability
- Reduced role strain

Independent living removes a significant source of cognitive and emotional load: constant negotiation. For many women, this results in a quieter internal environment and fewer emotional disruptions. Greater psychological clarity. A more regulated nervous system.

Cognitive Function: The Advantage of Mental Space
The brain requires uninterrupted time to integrate information, process emotion, and generate insight. Research on solitude demonstrates that intentional time alone supports (Nguyen et al., 2018):
- Cognitive flexibility
- Creative problem-solving
- Executive functioning
- Sustained attention

Without continuous external input, the brain engages in reflective processing. This allows:
- Better decision-making
- Stronger identity integration
- Increased clarity around long-term goals

Many women report that their most important insights emerge not in conversation, but in quiet. This is not incidental. It is neurocognitive recovery and optimization.

Resilience, Aging, and Longevity
Concerns about aging alone are often rooted in outdated assumptions rather than current data. Gerontological research consistently shows that women who age independently often demonstrate:
- Strong social integration
- High levels of adaptability
- Continued engagement in meaningful activities
- Preserved functional independence (Antonucci et al., 2014; Dixon, 2020)

Longevity is most strongly associated with social connection, purpose, and behavioral health patterns. Not marital status (Holt-Lunstad et al., 2010). In fact, distributed social networks, rather than reliance on a single partner, often provide greater resilience over time.

Identity, Self-Efficacy, and Health Behavior
Perhaps the most significant health advantage of solo living is not physical. It is psychological. A self-directed life strengthens self-efficacy, defined as the belief in one's ability to manage life effectively (Bandura, 1997). High self-efficacy is associated with:
- Lower anxiety and depression
- Greater adherence to health behaviors
- Improved coping under stress
- Better long-term health outcomes

Single women develop self-efficacy through lived experience: Managing finances, navigating challenges independently, making complex decisions, and maintaining personal environments.

Each successful action reinforces a core belief: I can take care of my life. That belief is not abstract. It is biologically protective.

Health as Alignment
Across disciplines, a consistent pattern emerges. Health is optimized when life reflects autonomy, emotional regulation, meaningful connection, purpose, behavioral consistency, and supportive environments.

These conditions are not exclusive to singlehood. However, singlehood often provides a uniquely efficient structure for cultivating them. Independent living is not inherently a risk factor. It is a context. When approached intentionally, it becomes a powerful platform for health optimization.

A Reframed Understanding
The question is no longer: *"Is being single healthy?"* The more precise question is: *"Is the way I am living aligned with what supports my health?"*

When the answer is yes, the outcome is clear: Greater stability, stronger resilience, improved physical health, enhanced emotional well-being. A self-directed life does not guarantee health. It makes it more attainable.

The Body Responds to How You Live
Your body does not measure your life by relationship status. It responds to how you live it. To your routines. To your stress levels. To your sense of control. To your environment. To your relationships in all their forms.

When your life is aligned, your body reflects that alignment. This is the quiet advantage of solo living. Not absence. Structure. Not isolation. Clarity. Not deficiency. Design.

Integration: Applying the SOLO Method
Use these exercises to recognize, evaluate, and release expectations that no longer align with your life.

1. Redefine Health
Write down your current definition of health. Then ask: *Is this based on external standards or internal experience? Does it reflect how I feel or how I think I should function?* Rewrite: *Health, for me, is...*

2. Assess Your Current Alignment
Reflect on your daily habits. Identify: Behaviors that support your well-being and behaviors that work against it. Then ask: *Are my daily actions aligned with the way I want to feel long-term?*

3. Make One Intentional Adjustment
Choose one area to improve this week: Movement, sleep, nutrition, or stress management. Commit to one small change: *This week, I will support my health by...*

4. Reflect and Reinforce
At the end of the week, write: *What improved your well-being? What felt misaligned?* Then ask: *Am I building a life that consistently supports my health?*

Chapter 10: Aging with Strength and Clarity

"Remember always that you not only have the right to be an individual, you have an obligation to be one."
— Eleanor Roosevelt, Former First Lady and Human Rights Advocate

---

Seeing Aging Clearly

Aging rarely announces itself in a single moment. It emerges gradually, often at the edges of awareness, in quiet questions that gradually take on more weight. *Where will you live in the years ahead? How will you maintain independence? Who will be present when life inevitably shifts?*

These questions are not signs of fear. They are indicators of awareness. They signal a transition from passive expectation to intentional design. It is where the future is no longer something abstract or uncertain. It becomes something you shape deliberately, grounded in evidence, guided by values, and supported by systems that sustain autonomy, connection, and long-term well-being.

For women who have lived independently, aging is not a disruption of identity. It is a continuation of it. Within the SOLO Method, this chapter extends Outlook by exploring how autonomy and intentional design support healthy aging.

Reframing Aging: Beyond the Cultural Narrative

For decades, aging, particularly for single women, has been framed through a narrow and often inaccurate lens. Cultural narratives have emphasized decline, dependency, and isolation, reinforcing the idea that independence becomes fragile over time.

This narrative is not supported by contemporary evidence. Research across gerontology and public health consistently demonstrates that aging outcomes are shaped far more by behavioral, psychological, and social factors than by relationship status alone (National Academies of Sciences, Engineering, and Medicine, 2020; World Health Organization, 2021).

Autonomy, purpose, and meaningful social connection emerge as the primary determinants of healthy aging. When these elements are present, aging is not characterized by loss. It is characterized by continuity. The same qualities that support well-being in midlife, self-direction, emotional regulation, and adaptability, continue to function as protective factors across later life. Independence does not weaken aging. When cultivated intentionally, it strengthens it.

The Role of Autonomy in Healthy Aging
Autonomy remains one of the most consistent predictors of physical, cognitive, and emotional health across the lifespan. It reflects the ability to make decisions aligned with personal values rather than external pressure or necessity.

Women who maintain autonomy as they age demonstrate higher levels of mobility, stronger cognitive functioning, lower rates of depression, and greater overall life satisfaction (Ryan & Deci, 2020; World Health Organization, 2021). This is often described as self-maintained autonomy, a sustained capacity for independent decision-making and daily functioning. For women who have lived single, this capacity is not newly developed. It is already well established. Years of managing finances, navigating life transitions, making independent decisions, and structuring daily life create a foundation that carries forward into later adulthood. Autonomy does not eliminate the need for support. It reframes it. Support becomes integrated by choice rather than driven by necessity. This distinction preserves dignity and reinforces stability.

Social Connection: The True Foundation of Aging Well
One of the most persistent misconceptions is that partnership is the primary safeguard against loneliness in later life. Empirical evidence consistently contradicts this assumption. The most robust predictor of healthy aging is not marital status. It is the presence of meaningful, high-quality social connection. Strong social ties are associated with reduced mortality risk, improved immune functioning, better cognitive outcomes, and enhanced emotional well-being (Holt-Lunstad et al., 2010; National Academies of Sciences et al., 2020).

For many single women, relational life is not concentrated in one partnership. It is distributed across a network of friendships, community ties, neighbors, and chosen family. This distributed model of connection is structurally resilient. It allows relationships to evolve without destabilizing the entire support system. In contrast, individuals who rely on a single primary relationship, particularly one marked by emotional distance or conflict, may experience greater isolation despite being partnered. Connection is not defined by status. It is defined by quality, consistency, and reciprocity.

Purpose as a Lifelong Stabilizing Force

Purpose functions as a central organizing structure in later life. It is not limited to career or traditional roles. It reflects a sustained sense of direction, contribution, and meaning. Longitudinal research demonstrates that individuals with a strong sense of purpose experience better cognitive functioning, reduced risk of dementia, improved emotional regulation, and increased longevity (Alimujiang et al., 2019; Boyle et al., 2009; AshaRani et al., 2022).

For single women, purpose is often internally defined rather than externally assigned. It is not dependent on socially prescribed roles. It evolves through engagement in activities that reflect personal values, intellectual curiosity, and a commitment to contributing to others.

Purpose may be expressed through teaching, mentorship, creative work, community involvement, or continued learning. It adapts as circumstances change, maintaining continuity even as specific roles shift.
When purpose is internally anchored, it remains stable across transitions. It does not require validation to remain meaningful.

Health Behaviors and Independent Living

Patterns of daily living play a significant role in shaping long-term health outcomes. Evidence suggests that single adults, particularly women, often demonstrate strong health-promoting behaviors across the lifespan. Independent living allows for greater control over routines, including sleep, nutrition, physical activity, and preventive healthcare engagement (Umberson & Karas Montez, 2010; World Health Organization, 2021).

Without the cumulative strain of chronic relational conflict or disproportionate emotional labor, many women are able to allocate time and energy toward maintaining their physical and psychological well-being. Aging, in this context, becomes a process of refinement. Attention shifts toward preserving energy, minimizing unnecessary stressors, and supporting functional capacity. The body responds to consistency. It responds to care. It responds to alignment.

Designing for Long-Term Independence
Healthy aging is not only behavioral. It is environmental. The spaces you inhabit and the systems you create influence your ability to maintain independence over time. Research on aging in place emphasizes the importance of environments that support safety, accessibility, and connection (World Health Organization, 2021). This includes living spaces that reduce physical strain, communities that encourage engagement, and access to resources that support both health and daily functioning.

For single women, this represents an opportunity for intentional design. The future is not left to circumstance. It is structured through decisions made in the present. Aging well is cumulative. It reflects the integration of small, consistent choices that support long-term ease and stability.

Emotional Resilience Across the Lifespan
Aging inevitably includes change. Physical transitions, loss, and shifts in identity are part of the human experience. The determining factor is not whether these changes occur, but how they are navigated. Resilience is built over time through repeated adaptation. It reflects the ability to regulate emotions, reinterpret experiences, and respond flexibly to new circumstances.

Women who have lived independently often develop strong adaptive capacity. They are familiar with navigating uncertainty, making decisions without external validation, and recalibrating when circumstances shift. These experiences form a psychological infrastructure that supports stability in later life. Resilience is not an abstract concept. It is the accumulation of lived experience.

Rewriting the Narrative of Aging
The image of the vulnerable, isolated older single woman is not an accurate representation of contemporary life. It reflects outdated assumptions rather than current realities. Across communities, many single women are aging with strength, clarity, and intention. They remain socially engaged, cognitively active, and deeply connected to their environments and relationships. They do not experience aging as a diminishing of identity. They experience it as a deepening.

Autonomy becomes more refined. Boundaries become clearer. Relationships become more intentional. Purpose becomes more focused. Worth does not decline with age. It expands through experience, self-knowledge, and alignment.

Aging as a Continuation of the SOLO Framework
Aging is not separate from the life that precedes it. It is an extension of it. Within the SOLO Method, the same principles that guide midlife continue to shape later life: Sovereign remains the foundation of identity. Ownership sustains responsibility for choices and direction. Liberated expands connection beyond traditional constraints. Outlook ensures that the future is designed rather than deferred.

Aging with strength and clarity is not accidental. It is intentional. The question is no longer whether you will age. The question is how you will structure your life to carry you forward.

Practice: Aging with Intention
The following practices are designed to translate insight into action, reinforcing autonomy, connection, and long-term alignment. Begin by envisioning your future self. Imagine yourself in later life with clarity, stability, and independence. Consider where you live, how your days are structured, and who remains present in your life. This exercise provides a framework for present decisions.

Next, identify behaviors that support long-term autonomy. Focus on habits that preserve mobility, cognitive function, and emotional well-being. Small, consistent actions accumulate over time. Examine your current network of relationships. Consider which connections are strong, which require attention, and where new connections may be needed. Social structure is built intentionally. Clarify the underlying meaning within your current roles.

Purpose is not tied to a specific identity. It reflects deeper values that can be expressed in multiple ways across the lifespan. Evaluate your living environment. Identify adjustments that support both present comfort and future ease. Environmental design plays a critical role in maintaining independence. Reflect on past challenges you have successfully navigated. These experiences provide evidence of resilience and adaptive capacity. They serve as a foundation for future confidence.

Finally, consider what must be released and what must be protected to support long-term well-being. Aging with intention requires both. Each of these practices represents a decision. Each decision reinforces the structure of a life that is stable, aligned, and self-directed.

Integration: Applying the SOLO Method
Use these exercises to recognize, evaluate, and release expectations that no longer align with your life.

1. Redefine Aging
Write down your current beliefs about aging. Then ask: Are these beliefs based on evidence or cultural assumptions? Do they reflect limitation or possibility? Rewrite: *Aging, for me, is…*

2. Assess Your Future Alignment
Reflect on your current lifestyle. Consider: Health behaviors, social connections, and daily structure. Then ask: *If I continue living this way, what will my life look like in 10–20 years?*

3. Strengthen One Area of Longevity
Choose one area to intentionally improve: Physical health, cognitive engagement, social connection, and emotional resilience. Commit: *This week, I will strengthen my future by…*

4. Build Forward Momentum
At the end of the week, reflect: *What supported your long-term well-being? What needs adjustment?* Then ask: *Am I designing a life that will support me not just now, but over time?*

Chapter 11: When Silence Feels Like Doubt

When the Path Becomes Quiet

Every meaningful life includes seasons that feel less certain. Periods when momentum slows, external validation fades, and the future appears less defined than it once did. These moments do not signal failure. They signal transition.

For women who have chosen a self-directed life, these seasons can feel particularly pronounced. Without the constant reinforcement of traditional milestones, engagement, marriage, shared households, it becomes easier for doubt to surface. Questions may re-emerge, even after they have been resolved: *Is this still the right path? Would life feel easier if it looked more conventional? What will this choice mean over time?*

Within the SOLO Method, this chapter returns to Ownership by addressing internal doubt and strengthening self-trust in moments of uncertainty. Not the vision of the future at its clearest, but the experience of moving through uncertainty without abandoning alignment. Silence is not the absence of direction. It is the space where direction becomes internal.

Understanding Doubt as a Psychological Process

Doubt is often interpreted as a warning sign. In reality, it is more accurately understood as a regulatory process. From a psychological perspective, doubt functions as a form of cognitive and emotional recalibration. It emerges when the mind is evaluating whether current choices remain aligned with internal values, particularly during periods of change, fatigue, or reduced external feedback. Even well-established decisions can feel less stable under these conditions. This does not indicate that the decision has lost its validity. It indicates that the nervous system is seeking confirmation, clarity, or rest.

Research on self-regulation and identity development suggests that individuals who pursue non-normative life paths often experience periodic internal questioning, not because those paths are flawed, but because they lack consistent social reinforcement (Oyserman, 2009; Ryan & Deci, 2020). Doubt, in this context, is not a threat to authenticity. It is part of maintaining it.

The Return of the Cultural Script

Periods of quiet often amplify comparison. Not because your life is misaligned, but because cultural conditioning remains active. You have been repeatedly exposed to a specific model of adulthood. Partnership-centered, milestone-driven, socially validated. Even when consciously rejected, that model does not disappear entirely. It remains stored as a reference point.

When you encounter external markers such as weddings, anniversaries, or family milestones, that reference point can reactivate. The comparison that follows is not always a reflection of desire. It is often a reflection of familiarity.

Research on social comparison theory indicates that individuals evaluate their lives relative to perceived norms, particularly during periods of uncertainty (Festinger, 1957). When the dominant norm is highly visible, deviation can temporarily feel like misalignment, even when it is not. The critical distinction is this: Comparison reflects exposure. Alignment reflects truth.

External Voices and Internal Stability
Doubt is not always generated internally. It is often reinforced through subtle social interactions. Questions framed as concern, comments presented as humor, or assumptions embedded in everyday conversation can introduce friction. *"Are you still single?" "You'll find someone eventually." "Don't wait too long."* These statements are rarely malicious. They are expressions of inherited belief systems.

Repeated exposure to these messages can create what psychologists describe as identity-based pressure, where individuals feel compelled to align with socially validated roles despite internal misalignment. Maintaining stability in these moments requires a clear internal framework.

Your life is not evaluated by external narratives. It is constructed through internal alignment. Other people's discomfort does not indicate that your path is incorrect. It indicates that your path exists outside of their expectations.

Distinguishing Loneliness from Longing
One of the most important distinctions during quiet seasons is the difference between loneliness and longing. These experiences are often conflated, yet they reflect different psychological states.
Loneliness refers to a perceived lack of meaningful connection. It is associated with increased stress, poorer

health outcomes, and reduced emotional well-being (Hawkley & Cacioppo, 2010).

Longing, in contrast, reflects the presence of desire. It may involve a wish for deeper connection, shared experience, or emotional closeness, even within an otherwise stable and fulfilling life. Longing does not invalidate your choices. It provides information about your needs.

You may desire companionship without wanting to restructure your life around partnership. You may seek deeper emotional intimacy without abandoning independence. You may want shared experiences without relinquishing autonomy. When longing is misinterpreted as evidence of deficiency, it generates unnecessary distress. When it is recognized as a signal, it becomes actionable. The question shifts from: *"What is missing?"* to: *"How can I expand connection within the life I have chosen?"*

The Function of Quiet in Identity Development
Quiet seasons are not interruptions in the trajectory of your life. They are integral to it. Developmental psychology describes these periods as phases of integration, during which identity becomes more coherent and internally anchored. During integration:
- Previous beliefs are re-evaluated
- Emotional experiences are processed
- Priorities are reorganized
- Internal clarity increases

Without these periods, identity remains reactive. It is shaped by external input rather than internal reflection. Quiet creates the conditions for self-authorship to deepen.
It allows you to move beyond inherited narratives and refine your understanding of what is meaningful, sustainable, and true for you.

Inner Companionship as a Stabilizing Force
When external validation decreases, the relationship you have with yourself becomes central. This is where the work of previous chapters becomes visible. The autonomy you developed, the solitude you learned to navigate, and the self-trust you cultivated begin to function as stabilizing systems. Inner companionship reflects the ability to:
- Regulate emotional responses without immediate external input
- Interpret experiences with clarity rather than reactivity
- Maintain alignment despite temporary uncertainty

Research on self-compassion and emotional regulation indicates that individuals who respond to themselves with understanding rather than criticism demonstrate greater resilience, lower stress, and improved psychological well-being (Neff, 2011). Self-trust is not the absence of doubt. It is the ability to remain grounded even in the face of doubt.

Resilience in Nonlinear Life Paths
A self-directed life is not linear. It does not follow a predetermined sequence of milestones. As a result, it requires a higher tolerance for ambiguity. This tolerance is not a weakness. It is an adaptive strength.

Resilience research defines adaptive capacity as the ability to maintain stability while navigating change. Women who have built lives outside traditional structures often develop: Greater flexibility in decision-making, increased tolerance for uncertainty, stronger internal validation systems, and reduced dependence on external approval.

These qualities help you navigate periods of doubt without abandoning your broader direction. The absence of a predefined path does not create instability. It creates space for intentional design.

Reinterpreting the Experience of Doubt
The presence of doubt does not mean your life is misaligned. It means your life is being actively evaluated. When examined through a research-informed lens, doubt can be understood as:
- A signal of cognitive processing
- A response to reduced external reinforcement
- A reflection of exposure to dominant cultural narratives
- An opportunity for recalibration

Reframing doubt in this way removes its authority. It shifts it from a directive to a data point. You are not required to act on every thought that arises. You are not required to restructure your life based on temporary emotional states. Clarity is not achieved by eliminating doubt. It is achieved by understanding it.

Returning to Alignment
When doubt surfaces, the most effective response is not avoidance or immediate correction. It is reorientation. Return to the core question: *"Does this life reflect who I am and how I want to live?"* If the answer remains yes, even quietly, even without certainty, then the presence of doubt does not require a change in direction. It requires steadiness. Alignment is not loud. It is consistent.

Integration: Applying the SOLO Method
Use these exercises to recognize, evaluate, and release expectations that no longer align with your life.

1. Identify the Voice of Doubt

Notice a recent moment when doubt surfaced. Write: What triggered it and what thoughts followed. Then ask: *Is this doubt based on evidence, or is it a learned narrative?*

2. Separate Silence from Meaning

Reflect on a quiet or uncertain moment. Ask: *Am I interpreting silence as lack, or simply as space? What assumptions am I adding to this moment?* Then reframe: *This moment is not empty. It is...*

3. Distinguish Thought from Reality

Write down a recurring doubtful thought. Then separate: What is factually true and what is an interpretation. Ask: *What evidence supports this thought? What evidence does not?* This creates cognitive distance and reduces reactivity.

4. Emotional Regulation Check

Pause and assess your internal state. Notice: Physical sensations, emotional intensity, and mental clarity. Then ask: *Do I need to act, or to regulate?*

5. Re-anchor to Internal Authority

When doubt arises, return to your foundation. Ask:
- What do I know to be true about my values?
- What has already been clarified in my life?

Complete: *Even in uncertainty, I trust that...*

6. Interrupt the Narrative Loop

Notice if your mind is repeating the same concern.
Write: The thought and how many times it has surfaced. Then ask: *Is this problem-solving, or is this repetition?* Choose to pause the loop.

7. One Grounded Action

Choose one small action that reflects stability, not urgency.

This could include maintaining a routine, completing a simple task, or reaching out for connection. Afterward, reflect: *Did acting reduce doubt or reinforce it?*

8. Reinforce Self-Trust
At the end of the day, write: One moment where you navigated uncertainty effectively, and one decision you made without external validation. Then ask: *Am I learning to trust myself even when clarity is not immediate?*

Chapter 12: Unapologetically Single

The Moment You Stop Explaining

There comes a point on every self-authored path when explanation begins to feel unnecessary. Not because questions disappear. Not because judgment no longer exists. But because something internal has shifted. The need to justify your life quietly dissolves. This moment is not dramatic. It does not arrive with declaration or confrontation. It appears as a steady recognition: This life fits. No explanation is required.

Within the SOLO Method, this chapter reaffirms the Sovereign dimension by solidifying identity without reliance on external validation. Not as an idea, but as an embodiment. Identity is no longer negotiated. It is inhabited. You are no longer asking for permission to live this way. You are living it.

The Reality of Walking Outside the Script

A life that diverges from expectation will always invite attention. Sometimes curiosity. Sometimes admiration. Sometimes subtle or direct disapproval. These responses are not reflections of your life. They are reflections of the framework through which others interpret it.

Demographic data indicate that you are not alone in this path. In the United States, a substantial proportion of adults now live outside traditional couple structures, with many reporting high satisfaction, autonomy, and alignment with their chosen lifestyle (Fry, 2025). This is not an exception. It is a shift.

Yet cultural narratives often lag behind lived reality. As a result, you may find yourself navigating a social environment that has not fully updated its assumptions. Living unapologetically does not require correcting those assumptions. It requires no longer organizing your life around them.

Many individuals encounter a transitional phase in which external expectations remain psychologically active, even after they are consciously rejected. This creates a temporary form of cognitive dissonance. Behavior reflects autonomy, but internal dialogue may still echo inherited norms. This phase is not regression. It is recalibration. Over time, as self-directed choices are repeated and reinforced, internal congruence strengthens. The external script loses psychological authority not through resistance, but through disuse.

The Subtle Habit of Self-Reduction
One of the most persistent patterns among women living outside traditional expectations is not an overt apology but a subtle self-reduction. It appears in small adjustments: Diminishing accomplishments to remain socially acceptable. Softening opinions to avoid disruption. Downplaying independence to reduce discomfort in others. Redirecting conversations away from personal truth.

These behaviors function as micro-apologies. They are not spoken, but they are enacted. Over time, they create quite a distortion. Your life remains intact, but your expression of it becomes filtered. This filtering is not necessary. Your life is not excessive. Your clarity is not disruptive. Your independence is not a problem to be managed. The shift toward unapologetic living begins with recognizing where self-reduction has been normalized and deliberately choosing to withdraw from it.

This withdrawal is often incremental rather than immediate. It may begin with small acts of correction: allowing a statement to stand without softening, acknowledging an accomplishment without deflection, or maintaining a position without over-explanation. These moments may seem minor, yet they serve as behavioral realignments. Each instance reinforces a new internal standard. Over time, expression becomes more direct, less filtered, and more congruent with identity.

From External Validation to Internal Authority
A defining transition in psychological development is the movement from external validation to internal authority.
External validation asks: Am I acceptable? Internal authority states: I am aligned. Research on authenticity demonstrates that individuals who act in accordance with their internal values experience greater psychological well-being, emotional stability, and life satisfaction (Ryan & Deci, 2020; Wood et al., 2008).

This does not eliminate doubt or discomfort. It changes the reference point. Decisions are no longer filtered through anticipated reactions. They are evaluated through alignment. This shift is foundational. When internal authority is established, your life becomes coherent. It reflects your values rather than external expectations.
Understanding the Source of Judgment

Judgment is often misinterpreted as evaluation. It is frequently a projection. When others question your life, they may be expressing their own fear of independence. Their own uncertainty about alternative paths. Their own attachment to the narrative they have followed.

Research on social cognition indicates that individuals interpret others' choices through their own belief systems and emotional frameworks (Oyserman, 2009). Your life does not require translation to fit those frameworks. Not all discomfort directed toward you belongs to you. Unapologetic living involves recognizing this distinction and declining to absorb or resolve what is not yours to carry.

Boundaries as Structural Integrity
Living without apology requires boundaries. Not as defenses, but as structure. A boundary defines where you end, and others begin. It clarifies what you will engage with and what you will not. Healthy boundaries are consistently associated with improved mental health, stronger relationships, and reduced emotional exhaustion. When boundaries are established, a shift occurs: You are no longer managing other people's expectations. You are maintaining your own alignment.

Resistance may arise, particularly from individuals accustomed to previous versions of you. This resistance is not evidence of error. It is evidence of adjustment. Clarity stabilizes over time. Boundaries hold.

Allowing Yourself to Be Fully Visible
Taking up space is often misunderstood. It is not about dominance, but about presence without minimization and expression without qualification.
Research on self-expansion suggests that growth occurs when identity is fully expressed (Aron et al., 2013). When

you allow yourself to be visible, something shifts. You stop editing your life for comfort and translating your choices for acceptance. You become the central reference point of your life.

Strength Without Hardness
Unapologetic living is often mischaracterized as rigid or confrontational. In practice, it is neither. It is steady. It allows for warmth without self-abandonment. It allows for kindness without self-erasure. It allows for connection without compromise of identity. You can be soft and clear. You can be open and set boundaries. You can be generous and unwavering. This is not a contradiction. It is integration.

The Emotional Shift: From Justification to Ownership
The most significant transformation in unapologetic living is emotional, not behavioral. It is the movement from: *"I hope this makes sense to others."* To: *"This makes sense to me."*
From: *"I need this to be understood."* To: *"I am clear, whether it is understood or not."* This shift does not isolate you. It stabilizes you. When ownership replaces justification, your energy is no longer dispersed across explanation. It is directed toward living.

The Freedom of Full Alignment
When apology falls away, a different kind of freedom emerges. Decisions are made without rehearsing how they will be received, and rest no longer requires justification. What matters is pursued without minimization, and joy is experienced without restraint. This freedom is not impulsive. It is grounded in the recognition that your life does not require external approval to be valid. Alignment becomes the standard.

The Peak: Standing Fully in Your Life

Full alignment is not a fixed state. It is dynamic, evolving with growth, change, and new experiences. Periods of uncertainty may re-emerge, particularly during transitions, reflecting continued development rather than loss of progress. Psychological stability is not defined by constant alignment, but by the ability to return to internal authority when disruption occurs. At a certain point, often quietly, integration becomes clear. Not perfectly or permanently, but unmistakably. Nothing is missing. Nothing is waiting to begin. Nothing requires justification. The life being lived is intentional. From this position, what settles is not certainty in every outcome, but a steady certainty in oneself.

Integration: Applying the SOLO Method
Use these exercises to recognize, evaluate, and release expectations that no longer align with your life.

1. Define Your Identity Without Explanation
Write a clear statement of who you are, without referencing relationship status, roles, or others' expectations. Complete: *I am someone who…* Then ask: *Would I still define myself this way if no one were evaluating me?*

2. Release the Need to Justify
Reflect on situations where you feel the need to explain or defend your life choices. Write: *What you tend to say and why you feel the need to say it.* Then reframe: *My choices do not require explanation because…*

3. Practice Unapologetic Living
Choose one moment this week to respond differently. This may include not over-explaining your decisions, not softening your preferences, and not seeking reassurance. Afterward, reflect: *Did standing in my choices create discomfort, or did it create clarity?*

Chapter 13: The Life You Create

Beyond the Question of "What If"
At some point, the question changes. It is no longer: *Am I on the right path?* It becomes: *What do I want to build from here?* What remains is not a question of direction. It is a question of design.

Within the SOLO Method, this chapter integrates all four dimensions into a cohesive framework for designing a fully self-authored life. No longer as anticipation, but as active authorship. The future is no longer something to navigate. It is something you construct.

From Alignment to Expansion
Alignment stabilizes your life. Expansion evolves it. Once your life reflects your values, a new capacity emerges. You are no longer organizing your energy around correcting misalignment. You are free to extend, deepen, and build. Expansion does not require reinvention. It requires intention. You begin to ask different questions: *Where can this life grow? What has not yet been explored? What feels possible now that did not before?*

Research on adult development suggests that individuals who reach self-authorship naturally transition into a phase of self-transformation, where identity becomes more flexible, integrated, and future-oriented.

This is not a return to uncertainty. It is a progression into expansion. You are not starting over. You are building forward.

Designing a Life That Sustains You
A well-designed life is not reactive. It is structured. Structure does not limit freedom. It supports it. The most sustainable lives are built across multiple domains: Health that preserves energy and mobility, financial systems that support independence, relationships that reinforce connection and belonging, environments that reduce friction and increase ease, and purpose that provides direction and meaning.

These are not separate components. They function as an integrated system. When one area is neglected, strain appears. When all areas are intentionally supported, stability increases. Design is not about perfection. It is about coherence and sustainability over time.

Health as a Long-Term Investment
Health is not a short-term goal. It is infrastructure. The decisions made in midlife directly influence the quality of later life. Physical activity, sleep, nutrition, and stress regulation are not optional behaviors. They are foundational systems. Research consistently demonstrates that individuals who maintain consistent health behaviors experience improved functional independence, reduced chronic disease risk, greater cognitive longevity, and higher quality of life in later years (World Health Organization, 2021).

For women living independently, health becomes a form of self-leadership. You are not maintaining your body for appearance. You are maintaining it as a system that supports your continuity, independence, and long-term quality of life.

Financial Independence as Structural Freedom
Financial stability is not simply about security. It is about choice. The ability to make decisions without constraint is directly tied to financial autonomy. This includes not only income, but planning, investing, and long-term preparation.

Women who prioritize financial independence are better positioned to: Maintain control over living environments, access healthcare without delay, navigate transitions without crisis, and support their future selves with clarity. Financial systems are not restrictive. They are protective. They serve as the structural foundation that keeps your life self-directed over time.

Relationships as a Chosen Ecosystem
Connection does not diminish in importance as life evolves. It becomes more intentional. Rather than relying on proximity or default roles, relationships are deliberately curated, maintained, and expanded. A strong relational ecosystem includes Consistent friendships, community engagement, and intergenerational connection, shared experiences, and routines.

Research continues to confirm that diverse, high-quality relationships are among the strongest predictors of long-term well-being and longevity (Holt-Lunstad et al., 2010). Connection is not something that happens. It is something you actively design and consistently sustain.

Purpose as a Living Structure
Purpose is not static. It evolves. It is not tied to a single role, title, or identity. It reflects the ongoing expression of what matters to you. As life expands, purpose becomes more refined: more aligned with values, less dependent on external recognition, and more integrated into daily life.

Purpose provides direction without rigidity. It allows for continuity even as circumstances change. It anchors your life in meaning, even as structure evolves.

Environment as a Silent Architect

Your environment shapes your behavior more than intention alone. Spaces that are organized, accessible, and supportive reduce decision fatigue and increase consistency. Connected, engaging communities reinforce social participation. Environmental design is often overlooked, yet it plays a critical role in maintaining independence, supporting health behaviors, encouraging connection, and reducing stress (World Health Organization, 2021). Your environment is not neutral. It either reinforces your alignment or works against it.

Legacy: The Life That Extends Beyond You

Legacy is often misunderstood as something left behind. It is something that is lived. It is expressed through the way you treat others, the knowledge you share, the relationships you build, and the example you embody.

Legacy is not dependent on traditional roles. It is not limited to family structures or predefined pathways. It is created through consistency, presence, and contribution. The way you live demonstrates what is possible. You are not preparing for your legacy. You are already expressing it.

The Integration of the SOLO Method

At this point, the SOLO Method is no longer a framework. It is a lived system. Sovereign is your identity. Ownership is your behavior. Liberated is your connection. Outlook is your design. These elements no longer function separately. They operate simultaneously. Your life is no longer reactive. It is integrated.

The Final Shift: From Living to Leading

There is one final transition. You move from living your life to leading it. Not in a performative way. Not for recognition. But through quiet authority. You become: A model of self-trust, a reference point for alternative ways of living, and a source of stability for others navigating uncertainty. Leadership, in this context, is not about visibility. It is about embodiment.

The Ending That Is Not an Ending

There is no final destination in a self-authored life. There is only continuation. Growth continues. Adjustment continues. Expansion continues. What has changed is not the presence of uncertainty. It is your relationship with it. You are no longer waiting for life to begin. You are no longer measuring your life against someone else's timeline. You are no longer asking for permission. You are building.

The Final Truth

Nothing is missing. Nothing is late. Nothing requires correction. This life, as it stands, is not incomplete. It is intentional.

From this point forward, every decision, every structure, every relationship, every expansion reflects one central truth: This is your life. And you are fully capable of creating it the way you would like.

Integration: Applying the SOLO Method

Use these exercises to recognize, evaluate, and release expectations that no longer align with your life.

1. Integrate Your Framework

Reflect on the four components of the SOLO Method: Sovereign Ownership and a Liberated Outlook.

Ask: *How is each currently expressed in my life?* Identify one area that feels strong and one that needs refinement.

2. Define Your Life Structure

Describe how your life is intentionally designed today. Consider: Daily routines, relationships, environment, and priorities. Then ask: *Does my current structure reflect who I am, or whom I used to be?*

3. Choose Your Next Direction

Identify one area of your life you want to expand or evolve. Ask: *What feels aligned right now? What am I ready to build next?* Then commit: *The next direction I am intentionally moving toward is...*

4. Reinforce Ongoing Alignment

At the end of the week, reflect: What felt aligned and what felt misaligned. Then ask: *Am I continuing to build a life that reflects my values, or defaulting to old patterns?*

Conclusion

You Were Never Waiting

At the beginning, there was a question. A quiet one. Often unspoken. A question that lingered longer than it should have: *Is this it? Or am I still waiting for my real life to begin?* That question was never really about time. It was about permission. Permission to believe that your life, exactly as it is, could already be complete. Permission to trust that meaning does not arrive on a schedule. Permission to step outside a narrative that was never designed to hold the full complexity of who you are. This book has not given you a new life. It has helped you see the one you already have.

What Has Changed

Nothing about your external circumstances needed to shift for this realization to occur. What changed is how you interpret them. You no longer measure your life against a timeline that does not reflect your values. You no longer translate your choices into language that makes others comfortable. You no longer assume that something essential is missing simply because it has not followed a prescribed sequence.

You understand something now that is both simple and profound: Your life is not delayed. It is not incomplete. It is not waiting. It is happening.

The Quiet Reorganization

This shift did not require a dramatic reinvention. It happened in quieter ways. In the moment you stopped asking what you were supposed to want and began asking what fits. In recognition that connection exists in many forms, not just one. In the decision to trust your own voice, even when it stands apart from others. Over time, these moments created a reorganization. Not of your life, but of your meaning. What once felt uncertain became clear. What once felt missing became visible. What once required explanation became self-evident.

The Life You Are Living
You are not outside of love. You are within it. In friendships that are steady and real. In conversations that leave you understood. In the quiet presence of your own company. In the way you show up for others and for yourself. You are not outside of purpose. You are already expressing it. In the work you do. In the care you give. In the way you think, create, and contribute. You are not outside of meaning. You are living it. Not in one defining moment. But in the accumulation of days that reflect who you are.

What This Life Requires
A self-authored life is not easier. It is clearer. It requires you to listen more closely. To decide more intentionally. To tolerate uncertainty without immediately resolving it. It asks for something different than compliance. It asks for authorship. That does not mean certainty in every decision. It means trust in your ability to make them.

The Truth About This Path
There will still be moments of doubt. There will still be questions that resurface. There will still be times when the familiar script tries to pull you back into comparison.
That does not mean you are lost. It means you are aware. You now understand how to interpret those moments. You

recognize them as part of the process, not a signal to abandon it. You have learned how to return to yourself.

The Life That Continues
This is not an ending. It is a continuation. There is no final version of your life waiting to be reached. There is no moment when everything becomes fixed and complete. There is only ongoing creation. You will continue to: Refine what matters. Expand what feels aligned. Release what no longer fits. You will continue to build a life that reflects who you are becoming.

The Final Recognition
If there is one truth to carry forward, it is this: Nothing essential has been withheld from you. Not love. Not meaning. Not a possibility. What you were taught to wait for has been present all along. It was never located in a specific relationship, milestone, or outcome. It was located in you. In your ability to choose. In your capacity to create. In your willingness to live a life that reflects your truth rather than your expectations.

A Final Word to You
If that quiet question ever returns, and it may, you will know how to answer it now. Not with urgency. Not with doubt. But with clarity. This is not a waiting room. This is not a rehearsal. This is your life. And it is already fully yours.

Closing Reflection
There is nothing left to prove. Nothing left to be justified. Nothing left to wait for. Only something to continue: Living. Not as it was prescribed. Not as it was expected. But as it is chosen.

SOLO Method Self-Assessment

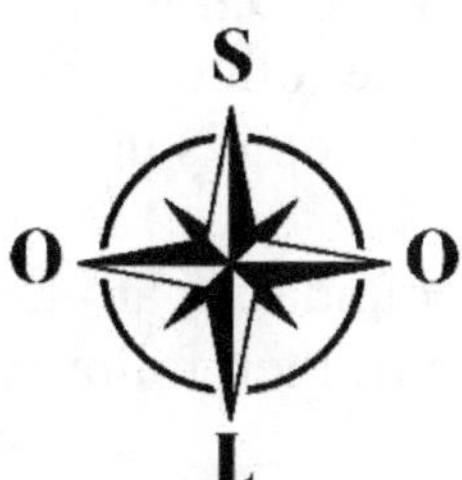

How Are You Thriving on Your Own?
Use this quick check-in to see where life already reflects the
SOLO Method, and where there is room to grow.

How to respond:
For each statement, circle a number from **1–5** that best
describes life in the past three months.
1 = Not at all true
2 = A little true
3 = Somewhat true
4 = Mostly true
5 = Completely true

S - *Sovereign*: Owning the Story
1. Life choices (work, home, relationships) reflect
   what feels right to you, not what others expect.
   1 2 3 4 5
2. You notice when old scripts about "should" appear
   and consciously decide whether they still fit.
   1 2 3 4 5
3. You feel comfortable describing yourself as single
   without apology or explanation.
   1 2 3 4 5

4. You protect your time, energy, and attention as if they are valuable resources.
1 2 3 4 5

O - *Ownership*: Designing Daily Life
5. Your daily routine reflects your actual priorities more than other people's demands.
1 2 3 4 5
6. You set clear boundaries around work, family, and social obligations, then follow through.
1 2 3 4 5
7. Money decisions (spending, saving, giving) line up with the kind of life you want in the next decade.
1 2 3 4 5
8. When something is not working, you create a specific plan to change it instead of waiting for circumstances to shift.
1 2 3 4 5

L - *Liberated*: Feeling Free in Your Own Skin
9. You feel more relief than anxiety when you remember that no partner has power over your daily choices.
1 2 3 4 5
10. You give yourself permission to enjoy pleasure, rest, hobbies, travel, intimacy, without guilt.
1 2 3 4 5
11. You rarely stay in situations (dates, friendships, obligations) that feel draining or disrespectful.
1 2 3 4 5
12. You feel free to show your real opinions, quirks, and preferences around people who matter.
1 2 3 4 5

O - *Outlook*: Building a Future That Fits
13. You feel more curious than afraid when you think about the next five to ten years.
1 2 3 4 5
14. You invest in your future self through learning, health habits, or new experiences.
1 2 3 4 5
15. You have at least a loose vision for later life that feels self-directed, not like a consolation prize.
1 2 3 4 5
16. You regularly nurture relationships (friends, family, chosen family, community) that support your solo life.
1 2 3 4 5

Scoring and Reflection
1. **Add your scores for each letter:**
    Sovereign (S): items 1–4, total 4–20
    Ownership (O): items 5–8, total 4–20
    Liberated (L): items 9–12, total 4–20
    Outlook (O): items 13–16, total 4–20

2. **Notice patterns**
    17–20: This area is a current strength. Life already reflects the SOLO Method here.
    12–16: This area is under construction. Small experiments could create big shifts.
    4–11: This area may still be shaped by old scripts, fear, or habit. Gentle attention here can change the story.

3. **Choose one next step**
    Look back at your lowest-scoring letter and pick one small, concrete action inspired by the practices in this book.

For example:
- S – Tell the truth in one conversation where you usually shrink or explain.
- O – Protect one evening each week as "off-limits" for obligations that do not nourish you.
- L – Say no to one draining invitation without offering a long explanation.
- O – Schedule one action that supports your future self: a class, a medical checkup, a money date, or a visit with a friend who feels like chosen family.

Place today's date at the top of this page and revisit the assessment in a few months. The goal is not a perfect score. The goal is a life that feels more sovereign, intentional, free, and open with each season.

References

Alimujiang, A., Wiensch, A., Boss, J., Fleischer, N. L., Mondul, A. M., McLean, K., Mukherjee, B., & Pearce, C. L. (2019). Association between life purpose and mortality among US adults older than 50 years. *JAMA Network Open, 2*(5), e194270. https://doi.org/10.1001/jamanetworkopen.2019.4270

Antonucci, T. C., Ajrouch, K. J., & Birditt, K. S. (2014). The convoy model: Explaining social relations from a multidisciplinary perspective. *The Gerontologist, 54*(1), 82–92. https://doi.org/10.1093/geront/gnt118

Aron, A., Fisher, H., Mashek, D. J., Strong, G., Li, H., & Brown, L. L. (2005). Reward, motivation, and emotion systems associated with early-stage intense romantic love. *Journal of Neurophysiology, 94*(1), 327–337. https://doi.org/10.1152/jn.00838.2004

AshaRani, P. V., Hombali, A., Seow, E., Ong, W. J., Tan, J. H., & Subramaniam, M. (2022). Perceived stigma and its association with mental health outcomes: A systematic review. *International Journal of Environmental Research and Public Health, 19*(3), 1230. https://doi.org/10.3390/ijerph19031230

Bandura, A. (1997). *Self-efficacy: The exercise of control*. W. H. Freeman.

Brake, E. (2012). *Minimizing marriage: Marriage, morality, and the law*. Oxford University Press.

Boyle, P. A., Barnes, L. L., Buchman, A. S., & Bennett, D. A. (2009). Purpose in life is associated with mortality among community-dwelling older persons. *Psychosomatic Medicine, 71*(5), 574–579. https://doi.org/10.1097/PSY.0b013e3181a5a7c0

Cialdini, R. B., & Goldstein, N. J. (2004). Social influence: Compliance and conformity. *Annual Review of Psychology, 55*, 591–621. https://doi.org/10.1146/annurev.psych.55.090902.142015

Demir, M., Özdemir, M., & Weitekamp, L. A. (2012). Looking to happy tomorrows with friends: Best and close friendships as predictors of happiness. *Journal of Happiness Studies, 13*, 101–119. https://doi.org/10.1007/s10902-011-9255-2

DePaulo, B. M. (2017). *Singled out: How singles are stereotyped, stigmatized, and ignored*. St. Martin's Press.

DePaulo, B. M. (2023). Single at heart: The power, freedom, and heart-filling joy of single life. *Psychology Today*.

Dixon, J. (2020). Loneliness and social isolation in older adults: A public health issue. *Journal of Aging and Health, 32*(5–6), 429–439.

Feeney, B. C., & Collins, N. L. (2015). A new look at social support: A theoretical perspective on thriving through relationships. *Personality and Social Psychology Review, 19*(2), 113–147. https://doi.org/10.1177/1088868314544222

Festinger, L. (1957). *A theory of cognitive dissonance*. Stanford University Press.

Fry, R. (2023). A record-high share of Americans have never been married. *Pew Research Center.*

Fry, R. (2023). *A rising share of U.S. adults are living without a spouse or partner*. Pew Research Center. https://www.pewresearch.org

Girme, Y. U., Overall, N. C., Faingataa, S., & Sibley, C. G. (2023). Singles are thriving: Evidence from a large population sample. *Perspectives on Psychological Science, 18*(3), 517–534. https://doi.org/10.1177/17456916221113228

Hawkley, L. C., & Cacioppo, J. T. (2010). Loneliness matters: A theoretical and empirical review. *Annals of Behavioral Medicine, 40*(2), 218–227. https://doi.org/10.1007/s12160-010-9210-8

Hill, P. L., & Turiano, N. A. (2014). Purpose in life as a predictor of mortality across adulthood. *Psychological Science, 25*(7), 1482–1486. https://doi.org/10.1177/0956797614531799

Hill, P. L., Turiano, N. A., Mroczek, D. K., & Roberts, B. W. (2016). Examining concurrent and longitudinal relations between personality traits and well-being. *Journal of Personality, 84*(2), 168–180.

Holt-Lunstad, J., Smith, T. B., & Layton, J. B. (2010). Social relationships and mortality risk. *PLoS Medicine, 7*(7), e1000316. https://doi.org/10.1371/journal.pmed.1000316

Kiecolt-Glaser, J. K., & Newton, T. L. (2001). Marriage and health: His and hers. *Psychological Bulletin, 127*(4), 472–503. https://doi.org/10.1037/0033-2909.127.4.472

Kim, E. S., Sun, J. K., Park, N., & Peterson, C. (2019). Purpose in life and reduced risk of mortality. *Journal of Behavioral Medicine, 42*, 123–133.

Long, C. R., & Averill, J. R. (2003). Solitude: An exploration of the benefits of being alone. *Journal for the Theory of Social Behaviour, 33*(1), 21–44.

Musick, K., & Bumpass, L. (2012). Re-examining the case for marriage. *Journal of Marriage and Family, 74*(1), 1–18.

Neff, K. D. (2011). Self-compassion, self-esteem, and well-being. *Social and Personality Psychology Compass, 5*(1), 1–12.

National Academies of Sciences, Engineering, and Medicine. (2020). *Social isolation and loneliness in older adults: Opportunities for the health care system*. National Academies Press. https://doi.org/10.17226/25663

Nguyen, T. V. T., Ryan, R. M., & Deci, E. L. (2018). Solitude as an approach to affective self-regulation. *Personality and Social Psychology Bulletin, 44*(1), 92–106.

Oyserman, D. (2009). Identity-based motivation: Implications for action-readiness. *Journal of Consumer Psychology, 19*(3), 250–260.

Park, Y., MacDonald, G., & Impett, E. A. (2022). Single and satisfied: A meta-analysis of relationship status and well-being. *Journal of Personality and Social Psychology, 123*(3), 567–589.

Reis, H. T., Clark, M. S., & Holmes, J. G. (2004). Perceived partner responsiveness. *Personality and Social Psychology Review, 8*(2), 155–172.

Ryan, R. M., & Deci, E. L. (2020). Intrinsic and extrinsic motivation from a self-determination theory perspective. *Contemporary Educational Psychology, 61*, 101860.

Sheldon, K. M., & Elliot, A. J. (1999). Goal striving, need satisfaction, and longitudinal well-being. *Journal of Personality and Social Psychology, 76*(3), 482–497.
Steger, M. F. (2012). Making meaning in life. *Psychological Inquiry, 23*(4), 381–385.
Umberson, D., & Karas Montez, J. (2010). Social relationships and health. *Journal of Health and Social Behavior, 51*(S), S54–S66.
Wood, A. M., Linley, P. A., Maltby, J., Baliousis, M., & Joseph, S. (2008). The authentic personality. *Journal of Counseling Psychology, 55*(3), 385–399.
Wright, M. R., Brown, S. L., & Manning, W. D. (2023). The health consequences of relationship quality. *Journal of Health and Social Behavior, 64*(1), 3–20.
World Health Organization. (2021). *Decade of healthy ageing: Baseline report.* https://www.who.int/publications/i/item/9789240017900

About The Author

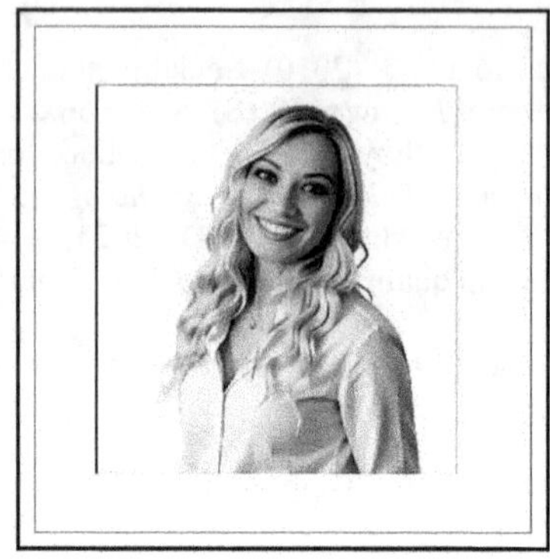

Dr. Tina M. Penhollow is a health behavior scientist, educator, and researcher with more than two decades of experience studying how individuals build meaningful, self-directed lives. Her work centers on autonomy, emotional resilience, purpose, and the alignment between identity and lifestyle.

Her research and writing challenge the long-standing narrative that fulfillment depends on traditional relationship paths. Instead, her work affirms that independence, particularly for women, reflects strength, clarity, and intentional living rather than absence or lack.

This book reflects that perspective. It offers evidence-informed insight and a reframing of what it means to live well, positioning autonomy as a valid and powerful life path.

Dr. Penhollow's work supports a growing cultural shift in which women define success, relationships, and identity on their own terms, grounded in authenticity, purpose, and self-trust.

Thank You!

Thank you for choosing this book and allowing these words to accompany you, even briefly, on your journey. Taking time to reflect and grow is an intentional act. It reflects a commitment to living with clarity, purpose, and authenticity. If these pages resonate, let them affirm this: your path does not require validation. Your life is already whole, as it is now. Meaning is created through how each day is lived. Let your time reflect what matters most: health, purpose, and alignment with your values.

With sincere gratitude,
- *Dr. Tina M. Penhollow*